**Practical Applications of Coaching
and Mentoring in Dentistry**

Practical Applications of Coaching and Mentoring in Dentistry

Janine Brooks

Dental Coaching and Training Consultancy
Dental Coaching Academy
Dental Mentors, UK

Helen Caton-Hughes

The Forton Group
Willoughby, UK

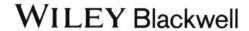

This edition first published 2021

© 2021 John Wiley & Sons Ltd

The right of Janine Brooks MBE and Helen Caton-Hughes to be identified as the authors of this work has been asserted in accordance with law.

Registered Offices
John Wiley & Sons, Inc., 111 River Street, Hoboken, NJ 07030, USA
John Wiley & Sons Ltd, The Atrium, Southern Gate, Chichester, West Sussex, PO19 8SQ, UK

Editorial Office
9600 Garsington Road, Oxford, OX4 2DQ, UK

For details of our global editorial offices, customer services, and more information about Wiley products visit us at www.wiley.com.

Wiley also publishes its books in a variety of electronic formats and by print-on-demand. Some content that appears in standard print versions of this book may not be available in other formats.

Library of Congress Cataloging-in-Publication Data
Names: Brooks, Janine, author. | Caton Hughes, Helen, author.
Title: Practical applications of coaching and mentoring in dentistry / Dr.
  Janine Brooks, Helen Caton-Hughes.
Description: First edition. | Hoboken, NJ : John Wiley & Sons, Inc., 2021. |
  Includes bibliographical references and index.
Identifiers: LCCN 2020045901 (print) | LCCN 2020045902 (ebook) | ISBN
  9781119648260 (paperback) | ISBN 9781119648222 (adobe pdf) | ISBN
  9781119648307 (epub)
Subjects: MESH: Mentoring | Dentists | United Kingdom
Classification: LCC RD37.2 (print) | LCC RD37.2 (ebook) | NLM WU 18 |
  DDC 617.0076–dc23
LC record available at https://lccn.loc.gov/2020045901
LC ebook record available at https://lccn.loc.gov/2020045902

Cover Design: Wiley
Cover Image: © (Top) Katja Kircher/Maskot/Getty Images;(Middle) Dean Mitchell/E+/Getty Images;
(Down) Sturti/E+/Getty Images

Set in 9.5/12.5pt STIXTwoText by SPi Global, Pondicherry, India
Printed and bound by CPI Group (UK) Ltd, Croydon, CR0 4YY

C103287_240321

Dedication

We would like to dedicate this book to all the hard working dental professionals who have successfully completed their post graduate qualifications in coaching and mentoring with Dental Coaching Academy. Their commitment to their profession, their own learning and development, and to coaching and mentoring has been an inspiration to us both, thank you.

Contents

About the Authors

Janine Brooks MBE, DMed Eth, MSc, FFGDP(UK), MCDH, DDPH(RCS), BDS, FAcadMEd, is CEO of Dentalia Coaching and Training Consultancy; Director of the Dental Coaching Academy; Co-founder of Dental Mentors UK; a private Coach and Mentor (Remediation, Career and Personal Development), Educational Associate and Registration Assessment Panelist for the General Dental Council; Trustee of the Dentists' Health Support Trust; Coach for the Professional Support Unit, Thames Valley; Expert Witness; Lead Clinical Tutor at the University of Bristol (BUOLD programme) and Honorary Fellow, Society of British Dental Nurses.

Janine enjoys a portfolio career working across a number of roles and organisations. Themes running through her work include education, mentoring and coaching. She launched my own coaching and training consultancy, Dentalia, in July 2011, providing coaching and mentoring to dental professionals and a broad range of education and training topics. She writes extensively and has published several books, plus a number of articles and papers over the years.

Helen and Janine along with their partner Bob launched a Post Graduate Certificate and a Post Graduate Award in Leadership Coaching and Mentoring in 2016. Over 60 dental professionals have successfully completed their qualifications to date.

Janine qualified from University of Birmingham dental school in 1983 and spent 19 years working as a Community Dentist in Herefordshire and Warwickshire before taking on national roles. Her main interests lie in bio ethics, professionalism, leadership in dentistry and mentoring.

Helen Caton-Hughes, MA, DipM, PCC, is an author, coach and founder of the Forton Group of companies. She combines her interest in health and wellbeing with leadership development and coaching. Her books include 'The Fertility Plan' and 'No Cape Required: empowering abundant leadership' (co-written with Bob Hughes).

Independent quality standards and a clear evidence base matter to her and Helen is an assessor for the International Coach Federation and a coach supervisor and mentor.

As a leadership, career and business coach, Helen works across the spectrum of health management, business development and marketing, with leaders from the private, public and humanitarian sectors and with their teams. Her clients include the UN, financial services and the UK National Health Service and leaders in fast growing technology companies, humanitarian organisations and logistics.

As a pioneer in digital business, Helen has built her own organisation based on flexible working patterns, digital technologies and self-paced remote learning. Equally at home in the classroom, Helen enjoys encouraging her students to discover their strengths, build their confidence and grow their careers as a result.

Helen's research includes youth volunteering, care home quality and the impacts of coaching on organisations. It's important to her that research findings get turned into actionable steps and, as a result, she designs training courses, including Post-Graduate programmes in leadership, coaching and mentoring, team-coaching and training in coach-mentoring and supervision. Helen also led the team that achieved the first International Coach Federation accredited programme to focus on leadership coaching.

Strongly committed to diversity, Helen works internationally, and inspired the development of abundant leadership, building on peoples' diverse strengths and talents, as well as their culture and values.

List of Contributors

Dr. Barkat Ahmed
BDS, CerMedEd, PGCert Dent Imp,
Diploma (Coaching and Mentoring)
Oxford, UK

Mrs. Shilpa Chitnis
BDS, PGCert Leadership Coaching and
Mentoring
GDP Practice Principal Coach Mentor
Andover, UK

Ms. Jane Davies-Slowik MBE
BDS- BDS MCDH DDPHRCS, PGCert
Leadership Coaching and Mentoring
Birmingham, UK

Dr. Stephen Denny
BDS, LDSRCS, PG Cert Dental Education,
PGCert Leadership Coaching and
Mentoring
Educational Supervisor; Honorary Tutor,
Southend Outreac; Clinical Educator
University of Essex
Southend, UK

Dr. Ahmad El-Toudmeri
Dental Surgeon, BDS
Sutton Coldfield, West Midlands, UK

Dr. Frederick Fernando
Dental Surgeon BDS PG Cert CMI
Saffron Walden, Essex, UK

Dr. Keith George
B.D.S D.P.DS, PGCert Leadership Coaching
and Mentoring
Burford, UK

Mrs. Sarah Jackson
BDS, PGCert Leadership Coaching and
Mentoring
Dental Surgeon
Poole, Dorset, UK

Mr. Sumair Khan
BDS (Lon) MFDS RCPS (Glas) MSc
(Implant Dent) Diploma (Rest Dent)
PGCert (Medical & Dent Ed) PGCert
(Leadership Coaching & Mentoring)
Training Programme Director - Oxford
Dental Foundation Training Scheme
Health Education England Thames Valley
& Wessex
Course Director - Postgraduate Diploma in
Implant Dentistry
Smile Dental Academy
Oxfordshire, UK

Dr. Claudia Peace
BDS, PGCert Leadership Coaching and
Mentoring
Dental Surgeon
Winchester, UK

Dr. Ewa Rozwadowska
BDS, PGCert Leadership Coaching and
Mentoring
Dental Surgeon
Cheltenham
UK

Dr. Catherine Rutland
BDS MA, BChD, IRMCert, CMI, BDS,
PGCert Leadership Coaching and
Mentoring
Clinical Director, Simplyhealth
and Denplan
Winchester, UK

Dr. Jin J. Vaghela
BDS (Lond) MFDS RCSEd (Edin) (London)
MJDF RCS (Eng) PG Cert (Dental
Education) FHEA PG Cert Leadership,
Mentoring & Coaching MSc Restorative
Dental Practice (Eastman)
DFT Educational Supervisor Health
Education East of England;
Visiting Lecturer Eastman Dental Institute;
Visiting Lecturer Royal College of
Surgeons;
Clinical Director Smile Clinic Group;
Clinical Director Smile Dental Academy,
London, UK

Foreword

When asked by the authors whether I would write a foreword to this book I felt hugely privileged. Having been trained in mentoring and coaching by them several years ago, their knowledge and passion for mentoring and coaching in dentistry should be written down to aid those of us who are always still learning.

The power of mentoring and coaching is still not fully used in dentistry. As I progress further though my career I see more and more the impact of what it can achieve. Whether in a formal setting, or supportive conversations within teams, it can really alter how individuals and teams progress and perform, ultimately leading to improved patient care.

This book and the methods it suggests are grounded in solid theory, and techniques and methods well tested and proven. The case studies within it show how mentoring and coaching can work in the real and often challenging world of dentistry.

It can be so easy to focus on clinical improvement within our development, yet there are so many other areas of our professional lives in which we can improve and work on. This can often get missed, yet a good mentor or coach will draw this out, ultimately leading to a more rounded and balanced career and, with that, a better work life balance and sense of wellbeing.

It is also important to recognise the joy and pleasure of being a mentor or coach, and watching people develop. Personally, that is one of the main reasons I worked for my qualification. I have been rewarded time and time again for the work required to achieve it, by seeing how you can support those who wish to engage.

Our careers can often take unexpected twists and turns, due to so many different factors, mine certainly has. Yet if you have someone to turn to who will mentor or coach you, depending on your need at the time, you find opportunities in the directions you can take and skills you may not have even known you had.

Enjoy this book and what it teaches you, and remember it is just the start of a bigger, and hugely rewarding journey.

Dr. Catherine Rutland
MA, BChD, IRMCert, CMI, BDS, PGCert Leadership Coaching and Mentoring
August 2020

Acknowledgements

We would like to acknowledge the kind participation and contributions of colleagues who generously shared the projects they have developed. Their projects have been included to help the profession to benefit from their experiences of introducing and using mentoring within dentistry.

Thank you to all our Case Study contributors: Dr. Barkat Ahmed, Dr. Jane Davies-Slowik MBE, Dr. Stephen Denny, Dr. Frederick Fernando, Dr. Keith George, Dr. Sarah Jackson, Dr. Sumair Khan, Dr. Claudia Peace, Dr. Ewa Rozwadowska, Dr. Catherine Rutland, Dr. Ahmad El-Toudmeri, Dr. Jin Vaghela, Dr. Shilpa Chitnis.

We would also like to thank our husbands, John Brooks and Bob Hughes for their unfailing support and encouragement, not to mention proof reading expertise.

1

Introduction

This book principally concerns itself with practical applications of mentoring within the profession of dentistry in the United Kingdom (UK). Whilst the book is written to showcase case studies within dentistry in the UK it is important to acknowledge that the skills of both dental professionals and mentors are not dissimilar throughout the world. If you are working outside the UK whether in dentistry or different field you will find much that you can take away from the book and the case studies. It is also important to acknowledge that whilst the case studies relate to dentists, their application is equally valid for all dental professionals.

The inspiration for the book came from students who have completed our post graduate certificate and award qualifications in mentoring and coaching. They are hard-working dental professionals with a passion for both dentistry and mentoring and we are indebted to their contributions. Future students will be directed to this publication as a course book, however it is not limited to being a course text.

We provide a number of case studies for projects which showcase how mentoring is being utilised in positive ways to enhance individuals and the services those individuals provide. The aim is to demonstrate how mentoring programmes can be implemented and the benefits they can bring. We invite you to submit your own case study examples to our website at www.dentalcoachingacademy.co.uk.

Whilst mentoring is a practical intervention it is underpinned by sound theory and the acquisition of mentoring skills. We have included chapters that describe mentoring and coaching as the two interventions share a number of skill areas, yet are quite different in purpose and application. We have also included a chapter on mentoring and coaching tools and models with particular attention to a model that we have successfully used in our training programmes. The discussion chapter will review topics that the case studies have introduced and other aspects that we hope will provoke further thought.

Please note: for readers outside the UK or those who are not dental professionals, organisations within the UK that relate to dentistry may read like alphabet soup. We refer you to the glossary for a brief explanation of the organisations and terminology used. Please also note that, unless we make specific distinctions, we use terms like 'coach' and 'mentor' interchangeably, as we hold no attachment to the terms in their general usage. If you want to 'coach' someone, that's great; if you prefer to 'mentor' them, that's fine too. Both are

Practical Applications of Coaching and Mentoring in Dentistry, First Edition.
Janine Brooks and Helen Caton-Hughes.
© 2021 John Wiley & Sons Ltd. Published 2021 by John Wiley & Sons Ltd.

possible as dental professionals supporting others' growth and development in general terms; or when we are acting as managers and leaders and drawing on coaching and mentoring skills generally. Where we make distinctions is when these skills are applied in professional settings and a precise tool, or approach is required by the context.

Mentoring is increasingly being seen by organisations generally, and the dental profession in particular, as a way of helping and supporting the development of people (employees, staff, contractors, patients) to achieve their goals. The word mentor has come to mean trusted adviser, friend, teacher, and wise person. The term 'coach' has been more commonly associated with someone supporting personal and professional performance, goal achievement, and drive. We aim to broaden both these terms to encompass enhanced self-awareness, development, personalised learning, and excellence in practise.

In dentistry we are still at the beginning of appreciating the potential and benefits of mentoring. In our experience more and more dental professionals are undertaking training to become mentors, such that these skills are applied more intentionally and more professionally. As will become evident as you read through the book, great mentors combine skill, expertise, and experience with the skills of mentoring in the service of another individual, the mentee. The practical skills, expertise, and experience that others wish to learn and emulate will not be covered by the book, they are taken as present. What the book does cover are the skills of translating that expertise and experience into a worthwhile, productive conversation, and relationship that promotes growth and development of another individual, the mentee.

History

Mentoring has slowly been gaining a position within dentistry since the Millennium with more and more dental professionals becoming familiar with the term and the concept of mentoring. It is also good to see this recognition from the statutory regulator for dental professionals.

> Activities such as coaching and mentoring, where individuals are supported by other members of the dental profession, also have an important role to play here, and are valuable ways of enhancing the skills and approach of all involved.
> Shifting the Balance: a better, fairer system of dental regulation (GDC 2017).

Vernon Holt did much to champion mentoring within the dental profession and his series of articles written between 2008 and 2010 are referenced frequently through the literature. Holt produced his thesis in 2013 and it contains a rich mine for those wishing to know more about mentoring in dentistry.

> I suggest that a culture proactively supportive of practitioners at all stages of their careers using routine mentoring could do more than any amount of audit of techniques, protocols or choosing of 'the latest' materials, to enhance the quality of care delivered. Furthermore, because the dentist has a leadership role in the practising

environment, the quality of performance of the dentist in the team can have a profound effect on the morale and culture of the team of which he or she is a part. This in turn will influence the quality of patient care indirectly as well as the direct effect through his/her own clinical performance (Holt 2013, p. 24).

It is from the 1980s that we start to see the emergence of a body of literature about mentoring in American business management (Colley 2002). Influential articles, particularly Roche's report, Much Ado about Mentoring (1979), claimed to have discovered mentoring as an informal but important part of a businessman's career. Mentoring in Britain then began to be seen as an American import, which had to be adapted to British culture. Clutterbuck was instrumental in the 1980s in bringing the idea of mentoring to Britain from the United States. He is regarded as the 'grandfather' of mentoring in the UK.

There is also anecdotal evidence to suggest that Continuing Professional Development (CPD) which involves interaction with professional colleagues has significant benefits when compared with other non-interactive activities, e.g. reading, or online CPD. While there is room for a mix of CPD activity, we all need to consider how to ensure that the benefits of interactive CPD are recognized and realised. Activities such as coaching and mentoring, where individuals are supported by other members of the dental profession, also have an important role to play here, and are valuable ways of enhancing the skills and approach of all involved (GDC Moving upstream 2020, p. 32).

Uses of Mentoring

Considering the widely varying circumstances and professional isolation of general dental practice, the most adaptable tool for supporting the quality of performance of dentists is likely to be mentoring (Holt 2013, p. 34).

Experience since Holt wrote the above sentence has shown that the potential for mentoring goes beyond quality performance. The case study examples in Chapter 5 highlight the following areas of benefit:

- Career development
- Quality assurance
- Improving communication
- Deepening insight and self-awareness
- Excellence
- Remediation of poor performance.

These are also explored further in the discussion chapter.

It's not only the dental practices that benefit from mentoring, the 2004 National Health Service (NHS) national staff survey (Healthcare Commission 2005) noted that 17% of staff identified that they had received training and development from a mentor during the previous 12 months.

The Department of Health, NHS knowledge and skills framework and development review (2004, p. 8) highlighted two key messages that relate to mentoring:

- Mentoring is key to the future of the NHS.
- A national framework for mentoring is to be created.

Viney and Paice (2010, p. 38) reporting on the London Deanery 'First Five Hundred' mentees concluded: 'The first five hundred mentees have confirmed our conviction that this service is needed and appreciated by a significate number of doctors and dentists'.

Increasingly, as clinical leadership grows, the use of mentoring and coaching to support leadership development is also growing. Many leadership programmes for health professionals now including a blend of training, development, mentoring, and coaching, as well as training for clinical leaders in mentoring and coaching skills.

Distinctions and Boundaries

As Clutterbuck outlined in 2001, there is considerable confusion over what mentoring is and what it is not. It can often be confused with other methods of professional support.

Here we make clear distinctions between counselling, advice-giving, coaching, and other 'talking' interventions. The distinctions focus on three key elements of mentoring:

- The type of support and level of advice that a Mentor gives a Mentee.
- The way in which support and advice is offered.
- The role(s) which the Mentee expects the Mentor to play.

For example:

- Counsellors tend to work with clinical issues and go back to the past before going forward. It's often a one-way relationship, with therapeutic intention.
- Mentors and coaches work with successful, healthy people and start in the present, then go to the future. In both cases, a two-way relationship is established – for example, mentors and coaches will share personal information and experience.
- Coaching encourages a partnership approach in the conversation, whereas a mentor, by dint of experience, knowledge, and connections, has greater perceived status and power than the mentee.

The divide between mentoring and coaching is less clear cut. Both work by encouraging self-discovery and self-resolution. A mentor is more likely to be an expert in the field and has been chosen because the mentee will look for advice and guidance from the mentor. A coach does not need to have any subject knowledge in order to produce results.

The range of skills or approaches used in mentoring may include training, advice, and career counselling. Understanding the distinctions between counselling, advice-giving, coaching, and other 'talking' interventions is important.

Advice-giving may include technical advice or business advice, and it's vital that mentors only give advice within the boundaries of their professional competencies and experience.

By comparison, a coach may offer examples from their own experience, but expect the coachee to use that example as a story or metaphor, for them to make sense of within their own context rather than as advice-giving.

This is not to set up either mentoring, coaching, or indeed any talking approach as 'better' or otherwise. Each has their role and benefits. The authors have been retained professionally as consultants, coaches, and mentors; their clients may, or may not, have been working separately with therapists or advisers. These are not competing modalities, rather they can be complementary. The mentee is an autonomous adult, capable of making their own decisions about what they need, and who they need to work with, in order to be personally and professionally successful.

Coaching and mentoring is also a style of leadership (Goleman et al. 2001) which can be summarised as a style of leadership that takes into account, and brings together what a person wants with the organisation's goals.

Table 1.1 A comparison of various interventions.

	Therapy	Mentoring	Consulting	Coaching
Focus of work	Deals mostly with a person's past and trauma, and seeks healing.	Deals mostly with succession training, and seeks to help the one being mentored to do as the mentor does	Deals mostly with problems and seeks to provide information (expertise, strategy, structures, methodologies) to solve the problems	Deals mostly with a client's present, and seeks to guide the client into a more desirable future.
Relationship	Doctor-patient relationship (therapist has the answers)	Older/wiser-younger/less experienced relationship (mentor has the answers)	Expert-person with problem relationship (consultant has the answers)	Co-creative equal partnership (coach helps client discover own answers)
Emotions	Assumes emotions are a symptom of something wrong	Is limited to emotional response of the mentoring parameters (succession, etc.)	Does not normally address or deal with emotions (informational only)	Assumes emotions are natural, and normalises them
Process	The therapist diagnoses, and then provides professional expertise and guidelines to give the client a path to healing.	The mentor allows student to observe mentor's behaviour, expertise: answers questions; provides guidance and wisdom for the stated purpose of the mentoring.	The consultant stands back, evaluates a situation, and then tells client the problems and how to fix it.	The coach stands with the client, and helps the client identify the challenges. Then they work together to turn challenges into victories. The client is held accountable to reach his or her desired goals.

Coach-like leaders and managers have conversations with their staff that go beyond short-term concerns, individual performance or team goals, and instead explore the person's life, including their dreams, life goals, and career hopes. This coach-like leaderships style has been identified as a key factor of better employee engagement (Engage for Success 2009), notably the 'Four Enablers' of engagement.

What's Inside This Book

Having outlined some key differences between interventions we can move onto think about how the book is structured.

Chapter 2 provides an outline of the mechanics of mentoring. This is an opportunity to consider the who and why of mentoring. The characteristics of mentoring and being a mentor are reviewed. We explore what mentoring can achieve and the different types of mentoring. There is a section on criteria that can help when choosing a mentor. The ethics of mentoring are also an important consideration in this chapter.

Chapter 3 reviews coaching: looking at what we mean by coaching, including definitions from the major coaching bodies. It also looks at some of the underpinning ideas or theories that inform coaching and which distinguishes this type of conversation from others, including differences between 'mentoring' and 'coaching'. This theory is applied through the practical skills covered in the following chapter.

Chapter 4 considers models used within mentoring and coaching with particular emphasis on the Forton model which is used extensively in our qualifications.

Chapter 5 is the key focus of the book, the case studies. Here we include 12 case studies generously provided by each of our contributors. The case studies are real examples of how to use mentoring practically within dentistry in the UK. The studies have been grouped into five categories which include: dentists in difficulty; evaluation; early years – undergraduates, foundation dentists, and post foundation; general practice; and organisational culture and models/tools. They showcase the diversity of using mentoring alongside mentoring tools and related techniques.

Chapter 6 covers discussion and conclusions. In this final chapter we review some of the lessons learned from the case studies and important themes that thread through. Communication is an aspect that can be found across the case studies and the categories of study. We look at some myths around mentoring and attempt to bust those myths. Looking beyond 1:1 mentoring is discussed as we consider team mentoring. Boundaries and barriers to mentoring also figure in the discussion and we conclude with a call for more case study contributions, to build on the body of knowledge, and with pointers for the way forward for coaching and mentoring in dentistry.

How to Use This Book

We invite you to apply choice in how you use this book! Some people like to read cover to cover, and the format also encourages dipping into a chapter at a time, depending on your preferred approach.

This is a 'text book', in as much as any book about coaching or mentoring can be; specifically for the post-graduate qualification programmes we teach. We also hope that dental professionals around the world will use this book as a starting point for developing their own skills and setting out on their own coaching and mentoring journey.

Inspiration is a personal experience, and yet we aspire to inspire. We hope this book will inspire you to find a coach or mentor, or to try out the coaching approach in your role as leader or manager or indeed to train to become a mentor or coach.

We also hope that you'll use this book to find out more about coaching and mentoring; we offer references at the end of each chapter and a 'Further Reading' list at the end of the book. We also invite you to get in touch with the authors, through the websites listed in the 'Further Reading' section.

References

Clutterbuck, D. (2001). *Everyone Needs a Mentor: Fostering Talent at Work*. Chartered Institute of Personnel and Development.

Colley, H. (2002). A 'rough guide' to the history of mentoring from a Marxist feminist perspective. *Journal of Education for Teaching* 28 (3): 247–263.

Department of Health (2004). The NHS knowledge and skills framework and the development review process.

Engage for Success (2009) https://engageforsuccess.org/the-four-enablers.

Gallwey, T., (1974) The Inner Game of Tennis. Joanathan Cape.

General Dental Council (2017). Shifting the Balance, A better, fairer system of dental regulation.

General Dental Council (2020). Moving upstream p.32.

Goleman, D. (2000). An EI-based theory of performance. In: *The Emotionally Intelligent Workplace* How to Select for, Measure, and Improve Emotional Intelligence in Individuals, Groups, and Organizations (eds. D. Goleman and C. Cherniss). San Francisco, CA: Jossey-Bass.

Healthcare Commission (2005). NHS national staff survey 2004 – summary of key findings.

Holt, R. (2013). Thesis, developing an holistic and person centred approach to professional practice and development using mentoring (with special reference to dentistry). Originally submitted for examination May 2013.

Holt, R., Ladwa, R., (2008). Mentoring. A quality assurance tool for dentists. Part 1: the need for mentoring in dental practice. *Primary Dental Care*. Oct:15(4):141–6.

Roche, G.R. (1979) Much Ado about mentors. *Harvard Business Review* [Online]. Available at https://hbr.org/1979/01/much-ado-about-mentors (Accessed 09 June 2020).

Viney, R. and Paice, E, (2010). The First Five Hundred. A Report on London Deanery's Coaching and Mentoring Service 2008–2010. The London Deanery.

Whitmore (1992). *Coaching for Performance: Growing People, Performance and Purpose*. Nicholas Brealey.

2

Mentoring

Holt and Ladwa (2008) in their study state that: 'The authors conclude that the best tool for supporting the quality of performance of dentists is mentoring'.

Such a short quote and yet it says so much and sets the tone for this Chapter. The key words are quality and performance, both should be interpreted as widely as possible.

In this chapter we will review the process and relationship that is mentoring. We will consider the roles and skills of being a mentor and what mentoring can achieve. There is a section on how to choose a mentor and some factors to think about when matching mentors and mentees. The important aspect of ethics is included. How supervision fits into mentoring and finally the current state of play in dentistry in the UK.

Mentoring is a relationship and a process, with a purpose: supporting someone to develop. It is a practical, applied activity, underpinned by skill and experience. Mentoring focuses on the present and on the mentees' future desired outcomes. The mentor supports the mentee to achieve those outcomes or goals, through a reflective, conversational process that combines their experience with their use of mentoring skills:

The magic of mentoring is the combination of insight arising in the mentee, inspiration, and motivation to take action toward a goal, and the confidence to keep going in the face of challenge.

For the magic of mentoring to happen both elements of skill and experience need to be present. It isn't enough to have expertise; it isn't enough to be great at listening, asking questions or developing rapport. A great mentor brings the two elements together in a harmony that is in service of the mentee and promotes growth and development.

In Its' Simplest Form the Mentoring Equation Is: Teacher + Coach = Mentor

The word 'Mentor' originally came from the Greek Classics – Homer's Odyssey. Mentor is a character's name; a person who teaches and oversees Odysseus' son, Telemachus. Mentor's cloak was a symbol of the protection his role provided Telemachus. In Greek Mythology, Minerva, goddess of schools, art, war and commerce, and, most importantly, wisdom, was also invoked.

Practical Applications of Coaching and Mentoring in Dentistry, First Edition.
Janine Brooks and Helen Caton-Hughes.
© 2021 John Wiley & Sons Ltd. Published 2021 by John Wiley & Sons Ltd.

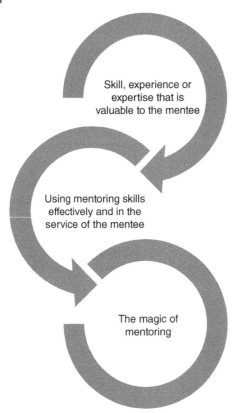

Figure 2.1 Experience + skill = mentoring magic.

Skill, experience or expertise that is valuable to the mentee

Using mentoring skills effectively and in the service of the mentee

The magic of mentoring

Combining these two powerful symbols creates a 'whole person': guided and taught externally, with inner wisdom and learning. Thus, mentor has come to mean trusted adviser, friend, teacher, and wise person.

The process of mentoring is defined in many ways:

> Off-line help by one person to another in making significant transitions in knowledge, work, or thinking (Clutterbuck and Megginson 1995).
>
> Mentoring is a developmental relationship where one person, typically older, or more experienced, or with more expert technical knowledge, shares their knowledge, skills, information, and perspective to support the personal and professional growth of someone else. In some cases, the mentor may also share their contacts or networks (Forton Group 2002).
>
> The process whereby an experienced, highly regarded, empathic person (the mentor), guides another individual (the mentee) in the development and re-examination of their own ideas, learning, and personal and professional development. The mentor who often, but not necessarily, works in the same organisation or field as the mentee, achieves this by listening and talking in confidence to the mentee (The Standing Conference on Postgraduate Medical and Dental Education SCOPME 1998).

Mentoring can be provided using a variety of formats. Face to face is perhaps the most frequently used, or there is distance/virtual mentoring using telephone or internet platforms where the mentor and mentee are in different locations, but it is still a one to one relationship.

Group mentoring is where a single mentor works with a group of mentees, for example within a dental practice setting, or via audio or visual conference facilities.

Who Is a Mentor?

The mentor is generally (although not always) a senior member of the profession who has a combination of experience, position, authority, and status. Regardless of seniority, mentors possess some experience, knowledge, and skills that are greater than the mentee.

Experience, knowledge, and skill acquisition is not age dependent and, in today's intergenerational workforce, less about older people mentoring younger colleagues (see Reverse Mentoring section).

The mentor uses their experience and attributes for the good of their mentee(s) in a positive and profitable relationship, which has the potential to benefit both sides. Blending roles for the benefit of the mentee takes training and experience.

The mentor may support their mentee to do a current job more effectively, offer insight into potential career paths or support the motivation or ambition of the mentee.

The mentor may have, and be willing to share, access to networks and connections, or have insights into personalities or relationships of potential value to the mentee.

The mentor may offer their knowledge and understanding of the structural, political, or social field of the workplace – both the visible and invisible structures – such that the mentee is better able to be resourceful, influential, and successful in that environment.

Why Be a Mentor?

Mentoring can be extremely rewarding, with huge satisfaction gained from seeing someone else learn and grow. It is a great personal development opportunity, compelling the mentor to think differently and more constructively.

Being a mentor will keep you on your toes, challenging you – like the child who keeps asking 'why?'. The beginner's mind-set helps experienced practitioners find new solutions to old problems. It gives insight into the way younger colleagues are treated and feel.

Reverse Mentoring

Reverse mentoring, sometimes called co-mentoring, refers to initiatives in which, for example, older individuals are paired with and mentored by younger individuals on topics such as technology, social media, and current trends.

In organisations that rely heavily on technology, reverse-mentoring is seen as a way to bring older colleagues up to speed in areas that are often second nature to younger people, whose lives have been more deeply integrated with digital technologies.

The idea that practice owners might learn from Foundation Trainees (FTs) goes against traditional professional practices, where more experienced dental professionals provide the most input, make decisions, and provide mentorship to newer professionals with less experience. Nonetheless, the fast-moving developments in technology, materials, and techniques in dentistry has reversed this logic; older professionals may have experience and insight, but lack skills in newer technologies and may not always recognise their potential.

Being mentored by a new colleague, takes a shift in attitude; it's an opportunity for give and take, where individuals share their knowledge, boosting everyone's understanding and improving overall communication and collaboration.

Reverse mentoring plays an important role in bridging intergenerational gaps: baby boomers (born between 1946 and 1964), Generation X (born between 1965 and 1976), and Generation Y, also called millennials (born between 1977 and 1996). A new generation is entering the workplace, Generation Z (born from 1997 onwards). In any one dental practice it will be commonplace to find four generations of dental professional working together. This will present both great opportunities and great challenges.

These groups have experienced vastly different social and cultural situations, resulting in varied work ethics, mindsets, and attitudes.

This has led to prejudices and stereotypes forming. For instance, some people view millennials as spoiled, unmotivated, and self-centered, while some millennials view older generations as inefficient and resistant to change.

Professionals need to learn how to cross the generational divide and communicate with, motivate and engage colleagues. Reverse mentoring challenges these stereotypes, and benefits team members, patients, and organisations alike.

Inter-professional Group Mentoring

This could be the most challenging mentoring format for some dental professionals to appreciate. This type of mentoring is when a mentor from one professional group, for example dentist mentors someone who is from a different professional group, for example dental nursing. Both mentor and mentee are dental professionals, however they undertake different roles. Whilst for some it might seem reasonable for a dentist to mentor a dental nurse and indeed it may be, the real challenge is when a dental nurse mentors a dentist. That may seem less reasonable. Or is it? This aspect of mentoring is covered within the discussion chapter.

The Roles of an Effective Mentor

The Mentor may help their mentee to do a current job more effectively, offer insight into potential career paths or support the mentee's motivation or ambition. In dentistry this is classically seen within the Educational Supervisor (ES)/FT/Vocational Trainee (VT) relationship. The mentor may have, and be willing to share, access to networks and connections, or have insights into personalities or relationships, of potential value to the mentee.

Many organisations and some practices that have mentoring programmes rely on the goodwill of senior dental professionals to volunteer their time. It's called 'giving back' to your organisation and to the profession.

Some great people mentor in this way, and their knowledge and experience is invaluable. However, there is no guarantee that such well-meaning volunteers will understand how to truly share all they have to offer or how to get the best out of their mentees.

The best mentoring programmes are based on formal training. That way, the mentor learns how best to pass on their wisdom and the mentee benefits from a more professional approach – a classic win–win.

The mentor may act at times as a teacher or adviser, or at other times more like a coach. The range of skills or approaches used may include training, advising, and career counselling. Understanding the distinctions between counselling, advice-giving, coaching, and other 'talking' interventions is important.

Mentors support mentees to explore their goals and provide the knowledge and experience to underpin their development. One key difference between 'teacher' and 'mentor' is that the teacher is an expert who shares information that they know with students, it is a one-way feed. In contrast, a coach may not be an expert or specialist in their coachee's field. They draw out solutions and clarity from the coachee, rather than put them in. Information sharing is not the coach's primary role. These differences are described in Table 1.1, Chapter 1.

Darling (1984) proposed a list of 14 characteristics and roles of an effective mentor:

- **Role Model** – Upholds high standards and professionalism. Well respected by peers whom the mentee 'looks up to' and holds in high regard. A powerful position of influence.
- **Envisioner** – Motivating, inspiring, and enthusiastic. Uses situations as opportunities to learn.
- **Energiser** – Keen to embrace change, improve care, and to encourage the mentee to see beyond the present and seek more.
- **Investor** – Gives their time, knowledge, and experience freely. Delegates responsibility to the mentee.
- **Supporter** – Willing to listen, encouraging. Humanistic and empathic in approach. Takes account of mentee anxiety and needs.
- **Standard prodder** – Seeks to improve standards. Demonstrates up to date knowledge.
- **Teacher-coach** – Passes on skills and competence, guides, sets up learning experiences, allows time for practice. Encourages personal and professional development. Provides and organises learning opportunities. Willing to share knowledge.
- **Feedback giver** – Gives constructive feedback, identifies future learning. Skilled questioner; facilitates reflection.
- **Eye opener** – Shows mentee the wider picture, e.g. politics, management, research.
- **Door opener** – Points out and brokers learning opportunities and resources.
- **Idea Bouncer** – Helps mentee reflect and generate new ideas, open to discussion and exploration of the literature.
- **Problem solver** – Helps mentee develop problem solving skills. Supportive when a mentee is struggling.
- **Career Counselor** – Gives guidance upon future directions and possibilities.
- **Challenger** – Helps mentee develop critically and encourages them to question and challenge views and prevailing norms.

Clearly a good mentor can be many different things to many different people. To what extent these roles will be utilised will depend on the issues a mentor is assisting their mentee with.

When mentoring for remediation the standard prodder role is important. When mentoring for personal development useful characteristics/roles are door opener, feedback giver, and idea bouncer.

Mentors have skills and qualifications and in particular skill-sets which, combined with their real-world experience of applying those skills, helps them to transfer that knowledge in a personal way.

For example, in dentistry a mentor may have business and commercial knowledge which, in combination with their clinical skills, offers insight into how to build a dental business.

What Can Mentoring Achieve?

Mentoring is a fruitful partnership at all stages of a dental professionals' career from the early days to preparing for retirement. Good mentors are independent, they support those who are struggling and guide personal development.

It can be hard to talk about your personal development needs with your boss, line manager, or even a trusted colleague. After all, they write your appraisal or debate your pay rise!

Finding a good mentor can be invaluable in improving confidence, providing insight, and identifying opportunities.

As Figure 2.2 below illustrates, mentoring can achieve benefits for the mentee, the mentor, for patients, and the whole organisation or practice.

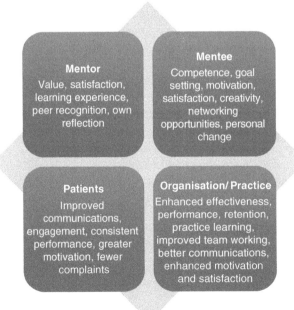

Mentor
Value, satisfaction, learning experience, peer recognition, own reflection

Mentee
Competence, goal setting, motivation, satisfaction, creativity, networking opportunities, personal change

Patients
Improved communications, engagement, consistent performance, greater motivation, fewer complaints

Organisation/Practice
Enhanced effectiveness, performance, retention, practice learning, improved team working, better communications, enhanced motivation and satisfaction

Figure 2.2 The impacts of mentoring.

Some advantages may at first sight appear intangible, yet they can all translate into financial benefits and a more sustaining working environment. Practices that promote mentoring typically have lower staff turnover. Dental professionals who are more fulfilled at work are more likely to perform at their best for more of the time. Patients will notice differences in communication and they are more likely to be better engaged with their own care.

Mentoring is a supportive conversation that will benefit individuals in:

- Personal development planning
- Career planning
- Professionalism
- Performance issues
- General patient issues
- Practice management
- Business development.

Mentoring accelerates growth – by building confidence, sharing advice, opening trusted networks, and development based on the insight and experience of what works – transferring that wisdom from one person to another.

It's not just the mentee who benefits from supportive conversations: mentoring brings huge personal fulfilment for the mentor.

Choosing a Mentor

The relationship between mentor and mentee is one high on openness and low on bias and ego. The relationship is essentially inter-developmental and the mentor should have no 'agenda'.

Trust is placed in the middle because it forms the core of creating a productive environment where relationship, words, and intention can flourish. Trust acts as the glue that binds everything together.

It is crucial to build a productive and equitable mentor/mentee relationship. The power of any working relationship lies not just in the strengths each individual brings, but also on equal input from both sides.

While the mentor may be someone with more experience, with greater knowledge, or senior to the mentee, it is important to acknowledge the capacity and potential of the mentee, in order to build equity.

The Power Relationship in Mentoring

Mentoring is not typically a partnership of equals: managing the power relationship issue is important for success. Yet a high degree of trust, openness, and mutual regard is vital.

The power relationship between mentor and mentee should **not** be too close. The mentor should **not** be the mentee's line manager. A mentor who is more than two levels above the mentee constitutes too great a power distance in which the mentee may feel uncomfortable.

It's important to see the role of mentor as being just one half of what will be a powerful relationship, where the mentor is as likely to benefit and develop through the process as does the mentee.

An imbalance of power carries with it the potential for abuse of the relationship or exploitation. 'Toxic mentoring' is a term that describes using mentoring in a negative way where the mentee, and sometimes the mentor, can suffer detrimental effects.

Compatibility and Rapport

Compatibility between the needs of the mentee and experience of the mentor is important. Getting on 'like a house on fire' is not necessarily effective in the longer term. The mentor must match compatibility with an ability to address the mentee's needs.

Coming from a mind-set of equal partnership can be effective in growing rapport.

When creating the mentoring 'contract' it's important to manage expectations, notably: the type of support and level of advice that a mentor is willing to give a mentee; the role(s) which the mentee expects the mentor to play.

When establishing personal and professional boundaries think about confirming the code of ethics and agreements that will underpin the partnership. Confirming the mentee's objectives and goals, will include: their current role; potential and future roles; networks and relationships; professional development requirements.

Diversity

This will include age, gender, culture, and ethnicity issues. Questions of diversity may be important: for example, in the mentoring of women, people from black or minority ethnic communities, or where religious, cultural, or sexuality issues may be relevant (within the current Equalities legislative framework). Each partner in the mentoring relationship should feel comfortable and able to identify relevant dimensions and express preferences on these issues.

Degree of Interest

The relationship needs sustained commitment over time, from both parties, to be successful.

Logistics

This includes geography and location, or different methods of contact such as face-to-face, telephone, email, virtual platform. It includes timing: how often mentor and mentee meet depends on how much time each are able to devote to mentoring, peoples' needs, and the mentoring objectives.

It is helpful to have mutual agreement on these points before the mentoring partnership begins.

Sanctions will also need to be thought about for example, what happens if the mentee fails to attend a meeting.

Personality

Avoid impossible matches, i.e. those which clearly would not work, for example working with your partner (either business or spouse). Avoid matching very similar people as it can be beneficial to match personality opposites. Opposites can get on very well and the ensuing dialogue is likely to be more stimulating and certainly more challenging! Some of the key skills of mentoring and coaching are receptive listening, adopting a non-judgemental attitude and supporting the mentee by challenging their current thinking. These are not the domain of specific personality types, neither 'strong' or 'introvert' personality types; rather they are learned skills, honed by practise. What this means is that, as long as the mentor is well-trained and suitably experienced, you don't need to worry about matching 'strong' personalities to ensure that they get 'enough challenge'. So-called 'quiet' people can be challenging too! It's also unwise to assume that 'strong' personalities don't need a sensitive approach or an empathetic listening ear.

The goal is to match people such that the mentee can express their hopes and fears to a receptive, non-judgmental person who will give them the appropriate amount of guidance and enhance their self-awareness, such that they take the right decisions for themselves, their professional development and their career direction.

Roles and Responsibilities

Managing expectations around roles and responsibility is also important. It will include setting clear expectations, such as that the mentee is responsible for creating their own results.

Starting, maintaining, and closing the relationship professionally will often depend on the needs of the mentee, their goals, and how quickly they wish to progress.

To be successful, expectations need to be matched with how much the mentor is able to give to the partnership. A mismatch can lead to failure.

Finally, the partnership duration and whether it is focused on specific goals or more related to ongoing professional and continuing development.

Matching Mentor and Mentee

Some organisations set up formal schemes for mentoring; others encourage informal matching methods. Networking and word of mouth can lead to successful mentoring relationships. Suggested matching criteria are given in the table below:

Table 2.1 Matching criteria and the issues they raise.

Criteria	Issue(s) raised
Power over mentee	The power relationship between mentor and mentee should **not** be too close.
	The mentor should **not** be the mentee's line manager.
	A mentor more than two levels above the mentee constitutes a power distance in which the mentee may feel uncomfortable.
Compatibility between the needs of the mentee and experience of the mentor	Most important criterion.
	Getting on 'like a house on fire' not necessarily desirable or effective.
	Harmony and ability to address the mentee's needs are both important.
Diversity issues, including age, gender, and ethnicity	Identify relevant dimensions and express preferences on them.
An indication of interest	The relationship needs sustained commitment over time, from both parties.
Geography and location	Methods of contact (e.g. face-to-face, telephone, email).
	Regularity of contact.
	Agreements and sanctions (e.g. failure to attend).
Personality	Avoid 'impossible' matches.
	Avoid matching very similar people.

Ethics

Successful mentoring relationship are built on solid ethical foundations. Ethical practice underpins mentoring.

Ethics describes standards of what is morally right and wrong, good and bad, that classify what people should do and how they should act.

It's about moral choices, the values that lie behind those choices, the reasons why people make the choices they make and the language people use to describe their choices.

Ethical behaviour in mentoring is focused on the ethics of the relationship between the mentor and mentee.

Coaches and mentors of South Africa (COMSA) (2015) have produced an ethics toolkit, which suggests four areas of potential legal or ethical problems for mentors. These are: Boundaries, Confidentiality, Competence, and Dependency.

Ethical behaviours will be very familiar to dental professionals: honesty, trust, integrity, compassion, respect, empathy. They are the behaviours we demonstrate in caring for and treating our patients.

Of course, mentoring is a reciprocal relationship, so it is just as important that the mentee maintains ethical behaviour toward their mentor.

Table 2.2 Ethical checklist, COMSA.

Boundaries	Am I clear about my boundaries and are they in line with my values and beliefs?
	Have I established my client's boundaries?
Confidentiality	Am I prepared/able to maintain complete confidentiality?
	Are there issues which may potentially require a breach of confidentiality? Have these possibilities been discussed? (i.e. in the case of law-breaking, abuse, or organisational requirements)
Competence	Am I fully aware of the requirements of the coaching assignment?
	Am I fully aware of the needs of my client regarding expected outcomes?
	Do I have the requisite skills, knowledge, and experience to be able to assist the client?
	Am I prepared to refer the client to someone who is more capable to help them, if the need arises?
	Do I need to refer to a supervisor to ensure that I am able to provide the necessary competence?
Dependency	Am I encouraging the client to extend the process unnecessarily?
	Do I discourage the client from forming a reliance on my input?
	Is there a clear determination of expected outcomes and a consequent end to the process?

Openness and transparency are ethical considerations, as is trust. Trust is the confident belief in and reliance on the moral character and competence of another person. It's a confidence that another person, in this case the mentor, will act with the right motives and in accordance with their professional norms. Mutual trust is vital to, and underpins, the mentor/mentee relationship.

Integrity can be demonstrated by soundness of judgment, reliability, and being faithful to moral norms. A lack of integrity can be manifest as, hypocrisy, insincerity, bad faith, and self-deception.

Confidentiality is important to the mentoring relationship. The mentee needs to know that their conversations will be held confidentially and that information will not be disclosed by the mentor to another person without the mentee's consent.

The mentoring relationship is subject to the same confidentiality as that between dental professional and patient. This means that only in very exceptional circumstances, for example where the mentee reveals behaviour that places patients or other persons at serious risk of harm would the mentor be legally and morally obliged to disclose information. Hopefully these type of circumstances would be rare.

Mentors are role models and they have a responsibility for ensuring that their behaviour is ethical. Beneficence means to act to bring benefit to another and the ethical mentor acts for the benefit of the mentee, in their best interests. They also act in a way that doesn't cause harm (non-maleficence').

Mentors must be careful not to make misleading claims about their competence, qualification, or accreditation as a mentor. Their behaviour at all times must be fair and without discrimination, showing respect for their mentee as an individual.

The philosopher Immanuel Kant (1724–1804) said that rational human beings should be treated as an end in themselves, and not as a means to something else. In terms of the mentoring relationship this means that the mentor should not treat the mentee or the relationship solely for their (the mentors') own gain.

The mentoring relationship can be a very close relationship with often personal and private information being shared. It's important that professional boundaries are maintained and not crossed.

This can include personal boundaries, but also conflicts of interest where either the mentor or the mentee uses the relationship to gain inside information or an unfair advantage over other people. Both the mentor and the mentee need to feel 'safe' that the relationship is about mentoring and not about something else, there must be no hidden agendas.

Supervision

Supervision is one of those words that is loaded with meaning. Unfortunately, supervision is not always viewed as a positive activity. Dental professionals generally do not like the idea of someone looking over their shoulder, viewing their work and judging them. Within mentoring the term supervision has a more benign, supportive, and developmental meaning. It also has an important qualitative element. Professional coaching bodies require coaches to undertake supervision.

The International Coach Federation (ICF) (2020) defines supervision as:

> ....a collaborative learning practice to continually build the capacity of the coach through reflective dialogue for the benefit of both coaches and clients. Coaching Supervision focuses on the development of the coach's capacity through offering a richer and broader opportunity for support and development. Coaching Supervision creates a safe environment for the coach to share their successes and failures in becoming masterful in the way they work with their clients.

Supervision should be undertaken by all professional mentors and coaches. Supervisors will be trained mentors and coaches who have themselves undertaken further training to be supervisors. A trained supervisor can help the mentor to challenge their own thinking looking for issues of bias, assumption, and unhelpful behaviours. Mentors can get into bad habits. Supervision can identify any unethical practices. It can also help the mentor to grow and develop their skill and capacity. It should be part of continuing professional development for all mentors and coaches in dentistry. In addition, training, and working as a supervisor will 'up your own game' as a mentor/coach.

Professional supervision benefits the mentor by building their confidence in their own practise, supporting skills development and reflective learning. It reminds the mentor to keep up with professional standards, the latest information in any specialist fields in which they practise and to go further, for example in exploring the theory that informs the field of coaching and mentoring.

Naturally, supervision for mentors and coaches is a strengths-based and developmental approach, using the mentor's own strengths and resourcefulness to underpin their growth and learning.

Supervision supports mentors in the dilemmas and ethical questions that accompany every situation; it enables us to identify and utilise the resources available to us as mentors. It also supports mentors to hear and take feedback on board – whether that comes from their own reflection, from the clients they work with, or from their supervisors. For the organisations that commission and employ mentors and coaches, supervision has a monitoring and quality control role in ensuring that mentors are fit to practise.

We deliver our own (accredited) coach-mentoring and supervision training programme which crosses the spectrum of these roles.

Dental Mentors UK is an organisation that was set up to support dental professionals who are also mentors. It provides continuing professional development for mentors which is a requirement of the General Dental Council (GDC) to keep updated in all areas of a dental professional's practice. Importantly it also provides supervision, both one to one and in groups, see www.dentalmentorsuk.com.

The Current State of Play

Having considered mentoring in a general sense we wanted to finish the chapter thinking about the actual state of mentoring within dentistry in the UK currently. In many ways mentoring has a good level of acceptance in the profession. The term is used frequently across a wide range of settings. There are mentoring programmes for dental students set up by Dental Schools and Universities; programmes provided by Dental Corporates; programmes supported by Health Education England (HEE) and Dental Deaneries. FT's and VT's are supported by ES's who include mentoring within their role. Practitioner Advice and Support Schemes (PASS) incorporate elements of mentoring and the GDC (2019) recognises the importance of mentoring. In addition, many of the specialist societies in dentistry operate mentoring schemes. This is all good news and encouraging for the future of mentoring.

However, these encouraging signs are tempered by the often loose use and application of the terms mentor and mentoring. It seems more often to refer only to the clinical dental experience of the individual providing the mentoring. There also seems to be a closer relationship with the role of teacher than coach. At the beginning of the chapter there is an equation: Teacher + Coach = Mentor, it seems that the teacher ingredient has overshadowed the Coach ingredient in the making of mentors in dentistry.

It is disappointing that acquiring a qualification in mentoring is seen as less important. There is training given and that is positive, but often this training is short, just a few days. It takes more to become an accomplished mentor. This lack of regard for formal training seems to undervalue the real skill of mentoring beyond simply the passing on of knowledge or clinical skills. Brooks (2018) makes these points in her article; let's get serious about mentoring.

If we as a profession and individuals do not get serious about mentoring, we run the risk of sidelining it or assuming anyone who is a dental professional can mentor any other. This type of 'amateur' approach will deprive everyone of the real benefits that can be gained from mentoring. A well-trained mentor can bring more financial benefits to an organisation or practice than any new piece of kit or any new technique. Mentoring is the skill that keeps giving and growing.

Conclusion

Mentoring is a powerful conversational intervention that brings lasting benefits to all those within the environment of dentistry. It is most powerful if practised regularly throughout a career. There is a specific skill-set that can be acquired by mentors that can elevate mentoring from a basic transfer of skills to a level of personal fulfilment and excellence for the mentee.

References

Brooks, J.A. (2018). Let's get serious about mentoring. *British Dental Journal* 224 (2): 72.

Clutterbuck, D. and Megginson, D. (1995). *Mentoring in Action – A Practical Guide for Managers*. Kogan.

COMENSA Code of ethics (2015) www.comensa.org.za/Content/Images/COMENSA_Code_of_Ethics_and_Conduct_2017.pdf

Darling, L.A.W. (1984). What do nurses want in a mentor? *Journal of Nursing Administration* 14 (10): 42–44.

Forton Group (2002): Professional Leadership Coach Training Programme Student Guide.

General Dental Council (2019). Shaping the direction of lifelong learning for dental professionals – discussion document. General Dental Council.

Holt, R. and Ladwa, R. (2008). Mentoring. A quality assurance tool for dentists. Part 1: the need for mentoring in dental practice. *Primary Dental Care* 15 (4): 141–146.

International Coaching Federation (2020). Coaching supervision. www.coachfederation.org. (accessed on 21.07.2020).

Kant, I. (1781) Critique of Pure Reason. Translated by J.M.D. Meiklejohn. The Project Gutenberg ebook (ebook 4280), July 2003. www.gutenberg.org

Standing Committee on Postgraduate Medical and Dental Education. (1998). *An enquiry into mentoring*. A SCOPME report. London: Department of Health.

3

Coaching

In this chapter we'll look at what we mean by coaching, some definitions from the major coaching bodies, and some of the underpinning ideas or theories that inform coaching that distinguish this type of conversation from others, including differences between 'mentoring' and 'coaching'. This theory is applied through the practical skills covered in the next chapter.

What Is Coaching?

Here are some definitions from the major international coaching bodies that underpin their definitions with competency frameworks and Codes of Ethics:

> . . .partnering with clients in a thought-provoking and creative process that inspires them to maximize their personal and professional potential.
>
> *(International Coaching Federation 2020)*

> Coaching is a facilitated, dialogic and reflective learning process that aims to grow the individuals (or teams) awareness, responsibility and choice (thinking and behavioural).
>
> *(Association for Coaching 2020)*

> Coaching and Mentoring: It is a professionally guided process that inspires clients to maximise their personal and professional potential. It is a structured, purposeful and transformational process, helping clients to see and test alternative ways for improvement of competence, decision making and enhancement of quality of life. Coach and Mentor and client work together in a partnering relationship on strictly confidential terms. In this relationship, clients are experts on the content and decision making level; the coach and mentor is an expert in professionally guiding the process.
>
> *(European Mentoring and Coaching Council 2015)*

Practical Applications of Coaching and Mentoring in Dentistry, First Edition.
Janine Brooks and Helen Caton-Hughes.
© 2021 John Wiley & Sons Ltd. Published 2021 by John Wiley & Sons Ltd.

Notice that the last definition conflates 'coaching and mentoring' into a single process, which we see as aligning with our equation, Teacher + Coach = Mentor where the coach/mentor guides the process, the mentor teaches from their own experience and the client focuses on what they want or need to learn and make their own decisions as a result of the conversation.

In this book we use the terms 'mentee' and 'coachee' to describe the learners in receipt of the mentoring or coaching processes and the 'mentor' or 'coach' as the 'givers' of those processes.

As well as thinking about the process, we can look at coaching from the viewpoint of the coachee; so, while the process may be consistent, there are many different approaches to coaching.

A review of the ICF website identifies the following approaches offered by accredited training programmes:

- Attention Deficit Disorder/Attention Deficit Hyperactivity Disorder (ADD/ADHD)
- Business/organisation
- Career/transition
- Creativity
- Executive
- Health and Fitness
- Internal
- Leadership
- Life vision and enhancement
- Personal/organisational
- Relationship
- Small Business
- Spirituality
- Therapeutic/alternative

The Forton model and approach (Hughes and Caton-Hughes 2019), (itself an accredited ICF programme: The Professional Leadership Coach training programme) is based on an approach to better leadership and management, summed up as:

> Supporting people to lead, succeed and achieve their goals, without telling them what to do, or doing it for them. (The Forton Group 2020)

This approach focuses on the autonomy and empowerment of people, indicating a shift away from a directive style of management (external locus of control) to an internal locus of control. Since coaching can be about an individual, a group or team, and about organisations or systems, the underlying assumption is that those groups can also exercise a greater level of self-sufficiency, as exemplified in agile working and 'scrum' approaches to operational delivery.

At a management or leadership level, coaching supports an individual to see what autonomy they have within their organisation, and where opportunities lie to make improvements, create and embed change and support their direct reports and teams to be successful.

Example | 25

The Forton model was created with a leadership and management focus, taking the whole system into account. In recognition of this increased autonomy, the definition of leader is also shifting: the Forton approach being one of abundant leadership 'being personally successful and enabling success in others', where leadership is about the individual, the team they lead, the wider organization, and leadership in society.

Abundant leadership also recognises the multi-generational workforce, the increasing gender, cultural, and ethnic diversity in the workplace; it's an approach based on tapping into the diversity of styles, approaches, and specialisms that are needed in today's world of work.

As well as diverse approaches to coaching, there are also a range of coaching models, tools, and approaches. These are addressed in the next chapter, along with the skills and competences needed by those who wish to coach others.

Purpose of Coaching

The coaching profession has grown in response to an unmet need: that of personalising and internalising learning away from a traditional 'telling' or directive style of teaching, towards learners accepting greater responsibility for their role in the learning process.

This, in turn, is both a pragmatic and a necessary response to the shift away from standard and traditional methods of production, based on hierarchical localised structures, towards a globalised, interconnected economy, where products and services are less tangible, less physical, and the creation of which is not suited to a directed economy.

When production or service methods are standardised, then education and learning can also be standardised. Where individual, or local group decisions and actions are needed for non-standard products and processes, then the education and learning needs to flex to those diverse needs. Indeed, the very nature changes, away from a facts-based approach to one where the key skills are about creativity. A shift from left brain to right brain thinking.

Example

For example: the steam sterilisation process in dental practices. The learning process is structured, and the practise of sterilisation needs to be carried out, in the same way, consistently, day after day. There are a number of key factors; with different approaches for wrapped and unwrapped instruments; there are mechanical checks for the efficiency and safety of the equipment and so on. Once the operator has shown understanding and learned the processes, along with any variations (e.g. for different types of instruments), nothing much will change, unless or until the equipment changes, or new requirements are brought in, for example.

But think about other elements of the dental profession: helping patients make life-enhancing choices; recruiting and retaining staff; investing in and introducing new innovations and technologies; identifying career options and making choices about which direction to pursue. Learning these skills doesn't just require understanding of the laws, rules, policies, and processes; they then need applying to different people in different situations.

We're living in an age of sudden change; shocks and uncertainty, which require complex decisions and the ability to move forward without all the information, or with ambiguous and conflicting information. This requires a more flexible approach to thinking, communicating, and acting; it requires the ability to inspire and motivate oneself and others, to get beyond challenges and still deliver high quality services.

The following quote is often attributed to Charles Darwin; whoever actually said it sums up the adaptability and flexible thinking that coaching offers the coachee:

> It is not the most intellectual of the species that survives; it is not the strongest that survives; but the species that survives is the one that is able best to adapt and adjust to the changing environment in which it finds itself. (anon)

Where mentoring can support people to make decisions by learning from the experience of others and from the past, coaching supports people to tap deeply into their own inner resources, to make sense of the world as it is today, and to make decisions in this volatile environment.

To support people, coaching helps to develop inner resources such as personal and professional reflection, resourcefulness, accountability, and personal responsibility; creating awareness, learning, and identifying options; and in external effectiveness such as making better plans, awareness of options, enabling better choices; considering how to – and when to – forward actions.

Another key purpose of coaching is the 'double-loop learning' (Argyris 1977) process: whether at individual, group, team or organisational levels, learning is not just a one-time experience, it's also a process of feeding that learning back into the system for wider, and longer term, benefits.

At individual level, learning 'how I learn best' increases my ability to learn more effectively; in fact, even the knowledge that there is not just one way I learn best is helpful. Learning how to do a process and then identify areas for improvement can speed up a process without 'cutting corners'. It can cut costs, reduce waste, time, and effort. When that 'double-loop' learning is fed back into an organisation, and becomes part of the sharing culture with colleagues, the return on investment in coaching is remarkable.

To summarise, coaching – in the Forton model – is a process that supports decision making based on current conditions and future objectives, forwards action and embeds learning in individuals, groups, teams and organisations.

Some Coaching Examples

- A coachee in a client organisation is identified in an innovative way for its suppliers to cut costs by sharing a storage facility. This provided two key benefits: reduced overheads (passed on to the customer) and improved collaboration between suppliers, which improved the supply chain and reduced error.
- Following coaching a manager introduced two types of virtual meetings each week for their direct reports, who each worked at different locations in the business. The first were chaired by him and included an element of directive leadership: communicating information;

setting goals, and deadlines, etc. The second were run by the direct reports, where the manager was not present. These meetings reduced the manager's travel to meet in person with these people by two to three days a week. Through the coaching the manager also identified that, when he did travel to the locations, his focus was on his direct reports more – with better quality and more personal interactions – than when he spent more time (and cost) travelling and trying to keep up with the other demands of his role at the same time.

- A coachee was asked about the impacts of coaching on her role and any impacts on the organisation: 'I took a decision that saved around £1m' was the response. By using the coaching method to work through a challenge concerning property refurbishment at several locations, the coachee found a way to avoid external legal fees.
- A sales manager struggling to meet his targets for the month used his coaching skills to meet with each of her salespeople individually. 'I was open about the challenge and tapped into their own motivations and commitment to the organisation. It was just a conversation, yet we reached our target, as a team, despite the challenging financial environment'.

Topics in workplace coaching range from creating a leadership vision to developing technical skills, addressing management skills in relationships (peer, direct reports, and relationships with senior leaders), preventing, addressing, and resolving conflict; stepping up to new responsibilities and new ways of working, away from the professional and technical role, to truly being the leader. Coaching also addresses personal topics such as health and fitness, finances, shared values and relationships, and personal development generally, all of which impact on the workplace.

Coaching might be described as enhanced communication skills that tap into inner resources, with the purpose of provoking creativity and innovative ideas; sparking collaboration and mutual support; enabling change and improvements. In the next chapter, we'll look at some of the key underpinning models that help explain how these approaches might work.

Distinctions Between 'Coaching' and 'Mentoring'

To sum up, mentoring is typically different to coaching in three ways:

- The relationship is between someone more experienced (in any given technical area, or within an organisation) sharing their relevant experience with another, less experienced person; from this we can infer that mentoring is more focused on experience from the past, shared with the mentee.
- Support typically takes the form of advice or information sharing, which may sometimes include 'door opening' to opportunities, networks or contacts.
- Topics are typically in the field of career development: the skills and experience needed to choose a career direction, start a new role, develop in that role; and how to overcome the likely challenges and hurdles that might be faced.

This is not to say that mentoring or coaching are intrinsically 'better' one than another or that these generalisations, above, are always true. Actual mentoring conversations will vary, depending on the experience and levels of training of the mentor, and their assumptions about their role. It is this flexibility of approach that gives the coaching or mentoring conversation its power; it's not constrained by specific learning points or pre-determined learning objectives.

Some people believe that coaching includes no element of 'telling' at all and yet the ICF competence of 'direct communication' contradicts this belief:

> Coach shares observations, intuitions, comments, thoughts and feelings to serve the client's learning or forward movement...without any attachment to them being right. (ICF 2020)

This is reinforced by the competence of creating awareness:

> Coaches questions, intuitions, and observations have the potential to create new learning for the client. (ICF 2020)

Both mentoring and coaching work by encouraging self-discovery and self-resolution. A mentor is more likely to be an expert in the field and has been chosen because the mentee will look for advice and guidance from the mentor.

A coach does not have to have any subject knowledge in order to produce results, because the goal is to evoke the coachee's own learning – which includes preferred methods of learning, discovery, and managing learning materials and handling the learning process.

Both mentoring and coaching have strengths and limitations and, while it is important to understand and maintain distinctions at this stage, in a developmental conversation both approaches may be relevant.

> Mentoring is a long standing form of training, learning, and development and an increasingly popular tool for supporting personal development.

Distinction from coaching:

> developing a person's skills and knowledge so that their job performance improves, hopefully leading to the achievement of organisational objectives. It targets high performance and improvement at work, although it may also have an impact on an individual's private life. It usually lasts for a short period and focuses on specific skills and goals.
>
> CIPD (2009)

Ideas that Underpin Coaching

Resources and Resourcefulness

A significant shift in thinking from problem-solving to resourceful thinking was initiated in 1987 in an article by David Cooperrider and Suresh Srivastva, following Cooperrider's doctoral dissertation 'Appreciative Inquiry into Organizational Life' in 1985. Appreciative

Table 3.1 The emotional intelligence quadrant.

	Awareness	Management
Self	Insight and self-awareness	Choice and self-management
Other	Social awareness	Relationship management

Inquiry, or appreciative inquiry (AI) as it's known, is a strengths-based approach and an AI method developed from it that has been absorbed into many areas of organisational and personal development, including coaching and positive psychology.

The Forton (2005) approach to AI is to support coachees to reflect on and discover inner and outer resources using the acronym 'PIES' (physical, intellectual, emotional, and social resources); see Chapter 4 for details.

Inner resources also include emotional intelligence (Daniel Goleman 1996), which also relates to more emotionally intelligent conversations and thus, relationships and people management. Emotional Intelligence is built upon four areas: insight and self-awareness; self-management; social awareness; and relationship management.

The recognition that coachees have resources, choice, and must self-manage is fundamental and based on self-awareness. From there it's a further step to build intelligence in interpersonal relationships, recognising that, while we can't control the choices of others, we can understand and empathise with them, and thus have an impact on our relationships with others.

Egan's "Skilled Helper" Model

The skilled helper model is summarised by Egan (1998) as 'managing problems and developing opportunities'. His model has three stages which can be summed up as: Exploring, Challenging, and Achieving.

Exploration can be twofold: the current situation and the desired state or goal.

- Challenging has the purpose of not accepting the current state as a fixed and immutable 'given' and orienting towards 'solving the problem' by exploring and supporting the coachee to see different perspectives and future options.
- The achieving stage is about action planning: goal setting, exploring options, risks and limitations as well as having first steps in place.

The aim of the 'skilled helper' is to enable the coachee to focus on results through achievable targets. This is often summarised as 'SMART' goals, that is 'specific, measurable, achievable, realistic (or relevant) and time-bound'.

The skilled helper model, while originally designed to support the counselling field, has a clear framework and helps focus coaching and mentoring on skills and ability, rather than abstract or theoretical principles.

There are, however, limitations with the skilled helper model: primarily in that it prioritises 'problem solving' – that is, that it primarily has a remedial function, rather than a developmental focus. This has had a lasting impact, particularly in the dental profession, where coaching and mentoring are seen as tools for 'Dentists in Difficulty'; that is 'failures'; people with problems.

Skilled helpers need a minimum level of this skillset, for consistent professional standards, to be used well within the dental profession and to understand its' limitations.

The ability for coaching and mentoring to 'develop opportunities' in the sense of meta-learning (double-loop learning) and breaking the cycle of "problem-solution" and into the paradigm of unlocking peoples' potential, needs greater attention and is addressed in the next chapter.

The Traditional Role of a Skilled Helper

What is the traditional role of a skilled helper? Buckingham and Goodall (2019) offer three theories that traditional mentoring and coaching have sought to realise.

1) *'The theory of the source of truth:* "You do not realize that your suit is shabby, that your presentation is boring, or that your voice is grating, so it is up to your colleagues to tell you as plainly as possible." (The Mentor)
2) *The theory of learning (empty vessel theory)* – "You lack certain abilities you need to acquire, so your colleagues should teach them to you." (The Trainer/Teacher)
3) *The theory of excellence:* "great performance is universal, analysable, and describable, and that once defined, it can be transferred from one person to another, regardless of who each individual is." (The Assessor/Teacher)'

> Research reveals that none of these theories is true. The more we depend on them, and the more technology we base on them, the *less* learning and productivity we will get from others.
>
> *(Buckingham and Goodall 2019)*

Buckingham and Goodall argue that we lack the objectivity to identify or assess others' abilities, transfer them to anyone and that, in our efforts to 'fix' other people, we prompt their fight or flight syndrome (feelings of being criticised and other strong negative emotions) – despite our best intentions.

By focusing learning on the learner's own goals, by revealing (to the coachee) and building on, their existing strengths the learner can discover, understand, and develop those areas of strengths into a personalised and unique level of excellence, rather than a level of excellence measured against a pre-determined framework.

This requires engagement with the thoughts, beliefs, and feelings of the learner, known as 'affective learning', which goes alongside understanding ideas and knowledge and then developing skills.

Buckingham and Goodall quote Richard Boyatzis who writes about the links between development and neuroscience, 'The parasympathetic nervous system. . .stimulates adult neurogenesis (i.e. growth of new neurons…), a sense of well-being, better immune system functioning, and cognitive, emotional, and perceptual openness'.

Coaching enables people to define what 'excellence' looks like for them, reflect on how they achieved that level and how to do more of it; as well as insight into what gets in the way of their success and what derails them.

Coaching can highlight patterns of habitual high-performance behaviours and support the introduction, achievement, and maintenance of new goals.

Buckingham and Goodalls's theory of learning might be summed up as 'recognise it (the pattern of behaviour that results in excellence), anchor it, re-create it, and refine it. That is learning'.

Martin Seligman (1991), the father of 'positive psychology', identified three key attitudes that hinder learning and development, as they relate to negative events. The attitude that the negative event is

- **Permanent**: 'it'll never change' – as distinct from 'it's just a setback'
- **Personal**: 'it's entirely my fault' – as distinct from "that was unlucky'
- **Pervasive**: 'this always happens to me' – as distinct from 'that was a one-off'

Shifts in attitudes, another effect of the coaching paradigm, means that coachees can build resilience and create a different future for themselves and their colleagues.

How Does Coaching 'Work'?

The above two theories of learning (Buckingham and Goodall's and Seligman's) seem to sum up both how coaching works, and what gets in the way of learning.

In terms of the broader issue about what impact coaching has, a recent ICF study (2019), by the ICF Research Department identified some validated areas worthy of addressing when reviewing a coaching programme.

They identified a series of questions about coaching, sufficiently valid as test questions. These (generalised) questions include creating new routines/habits and sustaining them; making progress towards, or achieving goals. The four key areas are: 'transformation', 'insight and awareness', 'sustainability', and 'goals'.

Transformation
- Coaching has transformed my life.
- Coaching has been a life-changing experience for me.
- Coaching has forever improved my life in a deeply meaningful way.

Insight & Awareness
- I had unexpected revelations as a result of my coaching.
- I obtained unexpected insights as a result of my coaching.
- Coaching helped me reflect on my current attitudes.

Sustainability
- I have sustained a new routine that helps me as a result of coaching.
- I believe I have created a permanent new habit as a result of coaching.
- I have been able to maintain the gains I made from coaching.

Goals
- Coaching was central to me achieving at least one of my goals.
- I achieved a goal as a result of coaching.
- Through coaching, I have made progress toward my goals.

This means that the impacts of a coaching programme can be measured in a consistent way through these self-assessment questions and, potentially, compared to other interventions (e.g. mentoring, teaching, on the job learning, etc.) to identify the optimum learning intervention for different situations, contexts and so on.

Conclusion

Coaching is a professional conversation that can change habits and support learning and development. Coaching is based on a different learning paradigm from traditional fixed learning aims and objectives, aiming towards evoking self-discovery and autonomy, based on current strengths. This leads towards future excellence.

Its role is highly relevant in today's uncertain and complex world, particularly in situations that need novel, local and/or individual solutions, and rapid, sustainable change.

References

Argyris (1977). Double loop learning in organizations. *Harvard Business Review* https://hbr.org/1977/09/double-loop-learning-in-organizations (accessed 4 November 2020).

Association for Coaching, 2020, 'What is coaching?' https://www.associationforcoaching.com/page/WhyCoaching (accessed 6th May 2020).

Boyatzis, R.E. and Jack, A.I. (2018). The neuroscience of coaching. *Consulting Psychology Journal: Practice and Research* 70 (1): 11–27. https://doi.org/10.1037/cpb0000095 (accessed 4 November 2020).

Buckingham, M. and Goodall, A. (2019). The feedback fallacy. *Harvard Business Review*, March–April, (pp. 92–101) https://hbr.org/2019/03/the-feedback-fallacy (accessed 4 November 2020).

CIPD (2009) Mentoring Factsheet: https://www.cipd.co.uk/knowledge/fundamentals/people/development/coaching-mentoring-factsheet (accessed 4/11/2020).

Cooperrider, D. and Srivastva, S. (1987). *Research in Organisational Change and Development*, vol. 1, 126–169. JAI Press.

DiGirolamo, J.A., Barney, M., Thomas, J., and Tkach, A. (2019). *Validated Set of Coaching Outcome Measures*. International Coach Federation (ICF).

Egan, G. (1998). The Skilled Helper: *A Problem-Management Approach to Helping*. Brooks/Cole Publishing Company.

European Mentoring and Coaching Council (EMCC), Competence Framework Glossary, V2, 2015, revised 2017; https://emccpoland.org/wp-content/uploads/2018/02/EMCC-quality-glossary-v2.pdf, accessed 6 May 2020.

Goleman, D. (1996). *Emotional Intelligence: Why It Can Matter More Than IQ*. Bloomsbury Publishing.

Goleman, D. and Boyatzis, M.K. (2002). *The New Leaders: Transforming the Art of Leadership into the Science of Results*. Little, Brown.

Hughes, B. and Caton-Hughes, H. (2019). *No Cape Required: Empowering Abundant Leadership*. Business Expert Press.

International Coach Federation (2020), definition of coaching https://coachfederation.org/findacoach (accessed 6 May 2020).

Lindsay J., The Forton Group, (2005). Professional Leadership Coaching Training Programme Student Guide.

Reynolds, M., (2017). Outsmart Your Brain: Outsmart Your Brain: How to Master Your Mind When Emotions Take the Wheel, Co-visioning.

Seligman, M. (1991). *Learned Optimism: How to Change Your Mind and Your Life*. Alfred a Knopf Inc.

4

The Forton Model

In this chapter we look at the skills, competencies, and processes behind a successful coaching conversation. We introduce the Forton leadership coaching and mentoring model (2005) and explore why we think this is a useful model for the dental profession.

We'll link them to the principles underpinning a coaching approach (explored in the previous chapter) and where they might also be successfully adapted for use in mentoring conversations.

We'll explore key principles that underpin coaching and mentoring ('The Principles'), the skills a coach/mentor needs to develop (The Skills); the conversation framework ('The Steps'); the context in which coaching/mentoring takes place and the relevance of the individual's place in that environment and the role of the organisation ('The Field').

Skills and Competencies of Coaching

Upskilling matters in coaching and mentoring because every conversation matters. Poor communication results in poor performance, confusion, and low morale.

Whether the subject matter is service delivery, customer relationships, performance improvements or addressing sensitive issues, good communication skills can make or break the success of that conversation.

Whether a conversation is defined as 'mentoring' or 'coaching', we believe that competency and professionalism matter. This means holding coaches and mentors to a given standard and helping them understand what makes for a better coaching or mentoring conversation.

The challenge is that many people believe they are already up to a high level of competency in this skill-set. If your colleagues, friends, and family tell you what a great listener you are; remark 'that's a great question' to you; thank you for being understanding and supportive, and for noticing your empathy – congratulations!

If however, you work in an environment of misunderstood intentions; are living with the unintended consequences of something you've said – or have someone tell you that 'you haven't listened to a word I've said', then welcome, you're in the majority.

Practical Applications of Coaching and Mentoring in Dentistry, First Edition.
Janine Brooks and Helen Caton-Hughes.
© 2021 John Wiley & Sons Ltd. Published 2021 by John Wiley & Sons Ltd.

Definition of a 'Skill'

> an ability to do an activity or job well, especially because you have practised it
>
> *(Cambridge Dictionary 2020)*

and

> a type of work or activity which requires special training and knowledge.
>
> *(Collins Dictionary 2020)*

Defining skills gives us a framework of abilities to do a job well: supporting others to achieve their goals, learn, and grow.

Core skills (called 'Key Skills' by the Qualifications and Curriculum Authority in England [QCA] and 'core skills' by the Scottish Qualifications Authority in Scotland (SQA, 2020) cover topics such as: communication, numeracy, information, and communication technology, problem solving, working with others and improving one's own learning and performance.

Coaching and mentoring others combines several of these skills. And yes, these skills are practised every day, but without the additional discipline of having them evaluated by others, they risk being used ineffectively in professional situations.

Definition of Competency

We need to know how to be effective in supporting others to achieve their goals; then learn to do it to an effective level. Competency frameworks provide a context within which, and against which, specific skills can be evaluated. For example, receptive listening may be valuable in many contexts, but within the coaching context, it plays an important and central role.

Definitions of competence include:

> An important skill that is needed to do a job
>
> *(Cambridge Dictionary, 2020)*

> Competence is the ability to do something well or effectively.
>
> *(Collins Dictionary, 2020)*

Therefore, the mentor or coach needs to learn both what those skills are and develop them to a level of success, as defined by an independent competence framework, which is regularly reviewed and updated, such as those defined by the International Coach Federation (ICF) (2020–2021).

Thinking about the ICF questions (described in the 'Coaching' chapter, above) that can validly assess that success, can the mentor or coach use their skill sufficiently well to support goal or habit setting, progress, achievement, and/or the sustainable maintenance of any change? Can they enable a coachee to develop insight and awareness? Can they support life-changing experiences?

It should be noted that while a 'life-changing experience' is a subjective, personal experience, 'insight' can be demonstrated more objectively, such as through reflective speech or writing, while goals or habits are objectively observable.

The Role of the Coach

A coaching conversation is one of partnership and co-creation; evoking the skills, experience, and knowledge of the coachee such that their learning and development is internalised, and decisions are taken from a foundation of both insight and inspiration, motivation, and optimism.

The ICF has defined a set of competences that a skilled coach must reach, at minimum level, to achieve their credentials, currently defined as 'Associate Certified Coach' (ACC); 'Professional Certified Coach' (PCC) and 'Master Certified Coach' (MCC). The ICF also trains assessors to identify behaviours (known as 'markers') that evidence these competences and thus evaluate coach performance (ICF 2020) in a consistent way.

Tools for Mentoring and Coaching

One of the challenges we offer all our students, whether dental professionals or not, is to consider how they will adapt and apply the skills and tools of coaching and mentoring, in their context. This builds upon the wider coaching philosophy of autonomy in decision-making, flexibility, and adaptability to the local context.

This is not a challenge with an instant answer. Many students take months to ponder this, while others know where they might start – such as coaching/mentoring within an organisation – yet still have a longer-term vision for their mentoring skills within their career.

Without identifying specific tools for mentoring in this chapter – as distinct from coaching – we do offer these points for consideration:

- How might the chosen tool impact on the power or status relationship between the coach/mentor and mentee?
- If so, in which way is the relationship impacted? Partnership and equity (in our definition) is more 'coach-like'; authority and status imbalance point to a mentoring role.
- How might other modalities (such as consulting, training, teaching, or counselling) benefit the mentee? Having clarity as to which 'hat' the mentor is wearing at any time and understanding the boundaries, is important for coaches and mentors.

The 2021 ICF Coaching Competences set out eight factors which summarise what embodies a 'coaching mind-set', which are:

1) Acknowledges that clients are responsible for their own choices.
2) Engages in ongoing learning and development as a coach.
3) Develops an ongoing reflective practice to enhance one's coaching.
4) Remains aware of and open to the influence of context and culture on self and others.

5) Uses awareness of self and one's intuition to benefit clients.
6) Develops and maintains the ability to regulate one's emotions.
7) Mentally and emotionally prepares for sessions.
8) Seeks help from outside sources when necessary.

It's interesting to note that 'coaching mind-set' combines a number of factors: a philosophy of learning (clients 'responsible for their own choices'); the active role of the coach in their own personal and professional development (e.g. 'regulate one's emotions') and the need to 'seek help' as necessary'.

Using these eight factors as a guideline for 'coaching', also enables a mentor to appreciate the distinctions between the two modalities and apply the tools in this chapter in ways appropriate to the mentee and their context.

The Coaching 'Journey'

Whilst it is a cliché in the tradition of talent competitions, or celebrity dancing on national TV, that we go on a journey to success and stardom, the journey metaphor is still valuable to understanding the value and method of coaching and mentoring.

The journey, as a metaphor, also highlights the importance to coaching of storytelling, analogies, metaphors, and the use of imagery in the coaching conversation. They are shortcuts to emotions; they enable us to explain ourselves, or order our thoughts, more easily and help our brains communicate more effectively.

In this chapter, we take the reader on a journey and we invite you to consider the process of taking a trip, say a holiday. Here's a quick overview of the coaching journey through the steps of the Forton coaching conversation model:

Purpose

1) We have a picture of what a great holiday looks like for us (Vision).
2) We justify our need for a holiday; this isn't just about having fun; we've worked all year for this break. We deserve it (Values).
3) We recognise that we need to prepare for our holiday, to be at our best; whether that's getting fit for a holiday activity; update our wardrobe; buy the books to read beside the beach (Ideal Self).
4) We negotiate with our family and friends to ensure there's something for everyone who's coming along (Leadership).

Reality

5) We take a look at the stock of sun-cream in the cupboard and check what's in and out of date (Resources).
6) We look at what we've saved towards the holiday already, and what we need in total (the gap).

7) We explore how we feel about the planned holiday: not just the anticipated pleasure, but managing the stresses of sorting out the work commitments – prior to going away, and catching up on our return (Emotional Intelligence).

Plan

8) We plan how we might fill the gaps in our resources, where we need to prioritise, and what we need to do to mitigate any challenges, such as getting cover at work.

Action

9) We take steps towards achieving our goals. We pack our suitcases, get the passports and tickets ready. We go!

Review

10) We check in with what's working and what's not working towards achieving our goal, and we adjust our actions to ensure we stay on track. For example, if the weather forecast for our chosen destination isn't living up to our expectations, we may have some choices to make – whether that's investing in an umbrella, packing an extra jumper, or cancelling a picnic. (Adaptability)

Yet coaching and mentoring isn't just about the actions and choices. It's also about the learning and development – of individuals, teams, and yes, families. So this journey isn't just about the places we visit, it's also about the inner journey of self-discovery and discovering how we impact on others.

In coaching we talk about 'forwarding actions and deepening learning'; it's doing and 'being'. Which is a far more fulfilling and rewarding experience than either activity alone.

This means there's a visible journey, for all to see, and an invisible journey – how we've changed as a result of travelling.

The Forton Model

The Forton Professional Leadership Coaching Model has its own metaphor: that of planets and orbits:

- Planet one: the steps of the coaching conversation.
- Planet two: the principles of coaching.
- Planet three: the Field, or the world of the coaches.
- Planet four: the coaching skills.

The Field has its own sub-orbits: resources and resourcefulness are so vital to the coaching conversation that they have a mnemonic – and their own metaphor – to help coaches remember to explore each area in the coaching conversation – PIES:

- **P**hysical
- **I**ntellectual
- **E**motional, and
- **S**ocial resources

PIES feed and nourish us; in British culture they are 'comfort' food: warming, and filling. We prepare our picnic before setting out: the food, drink, and other things we need for the journey to be successful. If we travel alone, our packing may be light; by contrast, taking a child can add a whole new dimension to our preparations!

By exploring the resources in our vision for success, we know what needs to be in place for that success to happen. By exploring the resources we already have available to us, we boost our self-confidence in our ability to succeed. We also more easily identify the resources we need – the gaps – that are currently standing in the way of our success.

As coaches, we explore the Field to identify where those resources are, who can enable access to them and who is a gatekeeper, withholding access.

In leadership, part of our role is to understand and navigate the Field, such that our team members have the resources they need to be, individually and collectively, successful.

It's important to note that this is just a model: a way of presenting steps and processes to make them easier to apply (Figure 4.1). In a real-life coaching conversation, the coach might blend a principle within a step, explore the field then go back to purpose. The model is not linear, nor is it prescriptive; the goal is for the coach to have a free-flowing conversation that supports the coachee to get where they need to, by drawing on any relevant element of the model.

Coaching Principles

Before we explore the skills needed in a coaching conversation, we need to review the underpinning principles of coaching and mentoring. In our journey metaphor, the principles comprise the inner journey. The principles set the foundation for a developmental conversation and go some way to explaining the 'why' of the skills. They also highlight who you are *being* when you coach, not just what you are *doing*.

Many development areas that coaches identify in their learning journey relate to the shifts in attitudes, or leaning fully into the principles, in support of their development.

Partnership

The ICF emphasises a coachee-centric approach and the role of coach as a partner in the coaching conversation. The coaching conversation: where the topic and direction are identified by the coachee, who is also expected to define measures of success for the conversation and to uncover the issues relevant to the topic.

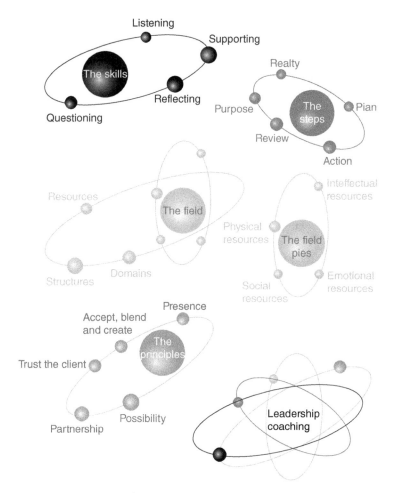

Figure 4.1   The Forton 'planets' model. Student Guide, The Forton Group, 2005.

This agreement creation (sometimes called 'contracting') is not a one-time discussion; it's an ongoing partnership. In the Forton model, we call this 'bookending and signposting' in the coaching; because, even if the coachee starts in a particular direction, or a goal in mind, that may shift as the conversation progresses and the role of the coach is to be led by the coachee in the direction they choose to go in. This doesn't mean that a coach may not challenge the coachee, or present options and different perspectives, but it does hold the coachee to be the expert in their own life.

The coaching conversations may have been preceded by a conversation about the overall direction or objectives of the coaching programme, to which others may have contributed. For example, the coachee's line manager, a member of the Human Resources or Leadership and Development team (sponsors) who may have a role in the coachee's development.

It is important to distinguish between the objectives for the coaching conversation and the content of the conversations themselves – the conversation itself remains confidential while the purpose or objectives may be known to others.

With well-defined objectives, it is then possible to measure both the outcomes and the impact of the coaching. The coaching conversation is only a catalyst for change; a precursor. Unless and until the coachee makes change in their inner world, coaching remains aspirational. Once change has happened, then the behavioural change is observable. The inner change is hard to observe, hence a better focus for success is to measure behavioural change: goal progress, achievement, and sustainability.

Whilst some coaching models start from the 'inside out', that is, they explore beliefs, attitudes, and values first, the Forton model is a behavioural one, that is, 'outside in'. This is not to say that it ignores the inner dimensions, far from it; it just means that it starts from a more tangible place, more easily accessible to a coachee.

The Forton Principle of Partnership is:

> Coaching is a relationship that requires both parties to trust, risk, and explore. To be most successful together, the coach and client should consciously work together to create agreements and structures that keep the partnership safe and effective. The ideal coaching relationship is purposeful, flexible, mutual, and sustainable.
>
> *(Forton 2005)*

Another way to look at the partnership is through the Forton Group 'Ask/Tell' Model:

In Figure 4.2, each mode describes certain roles. For example, when a new manager wants to establish her/his credibility s/he will share and tell what they know. This establishes trust that the manager knows what they're doing. However, if overused, it can lead to dependency and resentment – who wants to be told what to do the whole time? Traditional teaching, or sports coaching, are also examples of where someone who knows, tells someone who is new to the information, skill or knowledge.

More experienced managers ask questions of their team members; ask their opinions; explore options with them. This supports people to think for themselves and shifts

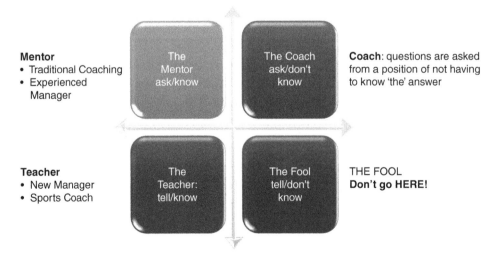

Figure 4.2 The Forton 'Ask/Tell' model. Student Guide, The Forton Group, 2005.

responsibility and accountability towards the team member. Likewise, with the mentor/ mentee relationship; asking questions, even from a position of experience and knowledge is a way to develop another person's sense of responsibility and accountability. And of course, there are times when a mentor will share their knowledge and information – by telling.

In 'pure' coaching the coach or mentor appreciates that they may not have 'all the answers'; that it's a good thing to withhold assumptions about what the 'right answer' might be. There might be more than one answer; an answer that used to be 'right' (or 'correct') may be outdated. With technology changing so rapidly, what was right yesterday, may not be the best answer today. Asking questions from an attitude of 'beginner's mind' or 'not knowing' can evoke some great ideas and innovation.

There's a time and a place for each of these three modes in the mentoring relationship, but hopefully no place for the fourth – the fool!

The 'Tell and Know' quadrant is a place where most people are comfortable to operate. This is a particularly comfortable mode for dental professionals who typically possess considerable knowledge and expertise.

The challenge for a successful mentor/mentee relationship is in moving to the 'Ask & Know' (ask questions, even when you might know some answers) and the 'Ask & Don't Know' quadrants (ask from a totally open perspective, with no assumptions as to the answers).

Principle Two: Trust

> The simple, often overlooked fact is this: work gets done with and through people. There's nothing more impactful on people, their work, and their performance, than trust.
>
> *(Covey 2006)*

In the Forton model principle of trust is based on a foundation of trust that the person being coached or mentored is capable, creative, wise and benevolent, and is acting with integrity. It doesn't mean they are infallible, or even necessarily trustworthy at all times in their life.

Students of coaching are expected to craft their own phrase to express this sense of trust, as they are shaped by our differing personal, cultural, and professional values.

The one most challenged by students is that of 'capability' – what if the coach doesn't believe their coachee is capable of what they aspire to?

This may be lack of trust in capability or potential capability, or it may be lack of belief in the coachee's potential: a subjective, limiting belief about another person.

The former is testable: if someone has the motivation to learn and the necessary resources to do so, then they will demonstrate their potential or actual capability – over time.

The latter may become a self-fulfilling prophecy: if they are not believed in and the coachee may not have the same access to resources that can enable them to achieve their potential. Therefore, trust in the coachee is an important principle of coaching.

What about 'earning trust'? This is another common misconception about trust: that it's a reward to be earned, rather than a gift to be given. Part of the maturing process is to shift to trusting one's own self: in decisions and actions, where previously we had trusted and relied on others. But that doesn't mean we withdraw trust in others as a consequence; it means that we know how, why, and when we can and can't trust ourselves and others. Just because someone 'fails' in one situation, doesn't mean we need to withdraw trust wholesale.

Trust is also an acceptance of our own fallibility, as well as the fallibility of others. When we trust ourselves and others we recognise those foibles.

We can also extend trust by seeing where a skill or talent is transferable: when someone can listen well in one situation, they are likely to be able to extend that skill to another.

These approaches to trust don't mean that our students have to accept these principles unthinkingly. This principle, in particular, demands that we reflect on our own beliefs about trust, and about notions of what 'success' and 'failure' mean to us.

The Coach Trusting Themselves

It is also important that the coach or mentor trusts themselves; their training, experience, and competence level as well as the value inherent in the process itself.

The mentor is likely to be making logical judgements based on the facts being discussed. They feel gut instincts: about the solution, about the mentee. Great mentoring comes from both the logical, tempered by the intuition.

Intuition is the way our brain has access to stored memories, it registers decision rules about what works and what doesn't; about how to deal with people, building on our feelings. This trustworthy experience store is the foundation of our intuition, repeated experience stored in the brain as memories without words, so that we can quickly access and interpret the signal our experience is trying to tell us.

That doesn't mean being wedded to the ideas or opinions that come from intuition. If the mentor senses their mentee is uncomfortable about something, we should ask them if that is the case. If they disagree, that's fine. Our intuition is never wrong – it is just sometimes misinterpreted!

Principle Three: Presence

Presence is about the quality of attention exhibited by a coach or mentor; someone who is focused and yet can respond in the moment to what the mentee is saying.

When fully-present a coach can listen more receptively; they are more alert to body language (without analysis or interpretation); they exercise self-control and remain calm, even in the midst of a challenging topic.

As well as exhibiting this calm demeanour, they are holding a responsive conversation, that holds the coachees' desired outcomes as an integral part of their overall focus. Holding back (or at least noticing, and then dismissing) judgement, they are responsive; partnering with the coachee and using their observational skills (responding to body language) as well as their listening skills.

Presence is built upon the ability to be calm and focused, to be silent when listening and stilling the busy mind. This often means that coaches will practise some form of mindfulness: whether visualisation, prayer, meditation or a physical practise like yoga or tai chi. They may take a few minutes before and after a coaching session to prepare for it, and to regain stillness afterwards.

Principle Four: Possibility

High-quality coaching and mentoring orients towards creating awareness of the many possibilities open to the coachee/mentee. It's not just about the problem or even the solution – great coaching digs deeper into the person, so they have the capacity to see different possibilities in the world and are hence equipped to resolve not just the problem they came with, but have learnt more about themselves through the process. Coaching and mentoring is not 'problem-solving'. This may sound paradoxical, but it's at the heart of the paradigm shift in learning that coaching has ushered in.

A problem is like a jigsaw puzzle. It has a single solution. Yes, some principles may be transferable to other puzzles: start with the edges, build from there; find an area of striking colour or detail that stands out, and so on. Yet part of the joy of puzzles is that they are all, in a satisfying way, alike.

The risk of being a listening ear to solving problems is that it creates a dependency on one person to another, whereas coaching and mentoring are about ensuring that the learner takes responsibility for discovering new solutions and applying them.

When the coach fixes one problem, the coachee will just bring more. When the coach focuses on the coachee as a person, they are focused on their development and on 'possibility'.

Today's world of work is beset by many challenges. Some entirely new. Some different. Some predictable. Some totally unexpected. While many principles can be learned and transferred from other sectors, countries or disciplines, what's possible may vary even within a single sector, or organisation.

To take this further, coaching isn't about 'the problem'; it's about the person, or the people in the team. When we help people to learn about themselves, discover their own possibilities and solutions, we enable them to gain maturity and self-reliance. This is truly empowering and is why there's a saying in coaching: 'coach the person, not the problem'.

This isn't to say that our coachees don't learn from teaching, advice, or research, but what coaching does is heighten awareness of the importance of both learning, and finding out how a coachee prefers to learn, such that they can explore what's possible, without the limitations placed on them by another's experience.

This is the 'double-loop' learning referred to in the previous chapter.

This is one point where the coaching journey differs from the mentoring journey: a mentor has a lifetime of past experience to offer; ways of doing things; expectations about who does what. In today's world, we need to explore how we might do things differently in future, and the coaching orientation towards possibility supports that.

A conversation that orients towards possibility is a significantly different conversation to one which solves a problem. Possibilities vary depending on the levels of resources, technologies, learning, and skills applied. So much more is possible than it was in the past. Holding an attitude of 'possibility' towards both the coachee/mentee and the goal towards which they are striving is a way of championing the individual, as well as supporting them towards their vision.

Principle Five: Accept, Blend, and Create (A, B, and C)

Another fundamental underpinning of the Forton coaching model is that of agility and spontaneity in the coaching/mentoring conversation. Sometimes known as the 'Bridge' technique, A, B, and C is a way to move the conversation forward towards the expressed possibility desired by the mentee – without getting stuck in the weeds of a problem, or negative attitudes.

A, B, and C is also inspired by the world of acting improvisation, often used in comedy. It's a flexible giving and receiving of ideas combined with spontaneity, and without a script. By trusting that someone in the group has the answer, everyone else can go with the flow of the situation, try things out and see what works, in a spirit of creativity.

- **Accepting** what the coachee/mentee says as being their truth, their reality, and not to judge or argue with it. We don't want to stay here. It's not permanent, personal or pervasive. There are ways to improve the situation. There is always possibility.
- **Blending** what the mentee offers as their current reality, with future possibility, is a way to offer new ideas – without attachment.
- This is a **Creative** moment. An offer could be a new way of looking at the situation. A new way of framing the challenge. A metaphor for the struggle. A fresh perspective. A challenging question.

The Principle of A, B, and C is underpinned by the belief that the role of coaching is to forward the action and deepen the learning in the mentee; not to stay with the problem or challenge, nor to try and 'fix' the problem. The 'fixing' approach is like throwing good money after bad. Focusing on the problem keeps us in the realm, or paradigm, of the problem. We don't want to be here and make things right with the problem; we want something new, better, and different.

This is not the same as ignoring risks, obstacles, or challenges. It's about ways to creatively neutralise those risks; re-frame the obstacle and overcome the challenge. Unlocking creativity supports innovation, improvements, cost savings, and the fulfilment that comes from approaching problems with a fresh pair of eyes.

The Skills of Coaching

The ICF takes the skills set and breaks it down into a detailed description of competences. The ICF have updated their competency framework over the years, as the profession evolves. To make it easier to start, the Forton model summarises four skills: listening; questioning; reflecting; and supporting. While the first three skills are used throughout the coaching or mentoring conversation, the fourth is like an armoury of specialist weapons, only used at key points in the conversation to encourage and support; to forward the action, and deepen the learning.

Receptive Listening

To be listened to well is a rare experience, and the impact can be immense. A mentor generates more trust from the simple act of listening than in any other way. Sometimes, people listen, just waiting for a gap to tell their story. Other times, people just listen to the words. 'Receptive listening' is about paying attention to the words and everything that surrounds them: the context in which the words are being said; the emotions behind them; the person's behaviour as they talk, the beliefs underpinning their statements.

As clinicians, dental professionals generally are good listeners, but we can switch onto auto pilot. So, when acting as a mentor or being mentored, it is extremely important to actively listen to what the other person is saying, to what they are really saying.

Receptive listening starts with being curious about the other person and wanting to know more about them. Mentors, when they are listening well, are waiting to hear the gold – what I mean here is the real nugget of the conversation.

This is what the mentee really wants to talk about and where they are looking to gain support and guidance. To listen for the gold, it helps to listen to the whole person, not just what they say, but their body language, their facial expressions, the exact words they use and the emotions they demonstrate.

Other things to listen out for include:

- Context
- Language use: repetition, emphasis, avoidance, tone
- Behaviours: normal and out of the normal
- Beliefs and values: the coachees' way of seeing the world

Responsive, active listening also means that the coach is comfortable with silence and with giving both themselves, and the coachee, time to think, reflect, and respond.

As well as being an active listener, receptive to what's being expressed, it is important to recognise different levels or locations of our listening.

- Are we listening solely to the other person, or are we also listening to our own experience at the same time?
- Are we listening because we're waiting for our turn to speak?
- Are we listening at all, or mentally constructing our shopping list?

Receptive listening with presence means that we're focused on the coachee/mentee, actively taking in the whole picture (a deeper level of listening) and being agile enough to reflect back their words, their body language or their silence, and bring these factors into the next question.

In the coaching journey, receptive listening is a key role of the coach: to be a listening partner; helping the coachee make sense and meaning from their own words – by firstly being heard, and then supporting the coachee to listen to themselves.

Asking Great Questions

When engaging in mentoring the questions we ask come from a place of curiosity rather than a place of knowing. To begin with stick to short open questions starting with: What?, Where?, How?, When?, and Who?. Open questions are important, these are questions that require more than just a simple yes or no as the answer. They open up the conversation.

Great questions are asked from an attitude of sincere curiosity, with an intention of the answer being meaningful to the mentee. Initial questions could recap the current situation or help the mentor understand the mentee's situation. As information is shared which both the mentor and mentee already know, it's time to move on. Remember – the purpose of asking questions is for the benefit of **the mentee's** learning, not the mentors. Great questions are 'clean' in the sense of being surrounded by silence, giving the mentee the opportunity to think, reflect, and answer in his/her own time.

Some ways of asking questions can prove to be unhelpful, for example:

WHY questions can be challenging and unless asked with the right voice tone and body language they can create defensiveness and the mentee may close down. 'Why' questions often have implicit criticism in them ('why on earth. . .?')

'Why' questions can always be rephrased into open 'what' questions (for example; 'what was important about doing that?')

STACKED questions are where we ask more than one question at a time. The difficulty is that the mentee doesn't know which to answer first. This is typically a symptom of over-eagerness on the part of the mentor. The remedy is to just ask a question and let it land. If it does, great; if not, pause, let it go and ask another!

Ask one question at a time and be comfortable with silence – mentees often use it for thinking and reflection time. Use it yourself; don't rush to ask a question. Take your time.

LEADING questions – 'have you thought about ...?' 'have you tried...?' – these are your answers! Leading questions are direction/advice questions given in a tone of voice that has a question mark at the end! Advice and information are better shared in a statement – phrased as a clear offer – which the mentee can accept, refuse, or adjust through reflection.

CLOSED QUESTIONS: Questions that require 'yes' or 'no' are great for clarifying **important** detail. Asking too many detailed closed questions runs the risk of directing the conversation to the mentors' ideas or solutions. When the mentor needs to gain commitment from the mentee to a challenge or setting up an 'accountability', closed questions can be helpful. As in 'will you do x by y'? The responses will generally be: yes/no/a renegotiate or a commitment to commit).

Yet a coach also needs to ask themselves, 'is a question really needed?' Coaches don't ask questions for the sake of being heard; they ask them to explore, test, and challenge; to re-focus on the coaching goal and to offer insights.

There's no rush to ask a question. Whilst fluidity is good and a natural, conversational style of coaching is more desirable than a forced or stilted question and answer session, sometimes the coach needs to take their time to formulate the question that begs to be asked.

The Skills of Reflecting

A good coach or mentor is like a mirror, reflecting the coachees' or mentees' world back to them – so that they see it more clearly: as it is, and as they want it to be. Sometimes a question arises from something the coach has heard – or seen – or, in some cases, sensed. These are all types of reflecting.

Reflecting skills take several forms:

- Reflecting the language used by the mentee back to them. To check their meaning, to check how they feel about what they've just said; to understand what's important about those words.
- Reflecting the tone: the impact it had on the coach/mentor.
- Reflecting the energy, pace or emotional content (or lack of) in what's just been said.
- Reflecting body language.
- Commenting on what's not said.

Acknowledgement is also a reflecting skill: acknowledgement of effort; acknowledgement of someone's feeling; acknowledgement of how challenging something might be.

Acknowledgement is about the effort of trying things out, reflecting on what works – and having the courage to acknowledge what doesn't. This is worth acknowledging for its own sake. Not necessarily because it's a success.

One of the most powerful acknowledgements is when we reflect back a quality we see in the other person – it might be courage, tenacity, compassion, or many others. Too often, we thank people for what they did, not for who they were being. Of course, it's important we do thank them, and there will also be times when the core quality is valuable to shine a light on.

When the reflecting skill is used well, people say they feel heard; they often comment on how nice it is to hear their words (sometimes as if they've heard themselves for the first time); and sometimes it gives them a chance to correct their meaning.

Reflecting requires the agility mentioned in the principle of coaching presence; the lack of attachment to what's said, and the understanding that it's the mentee or coachee who needs to understand what's really going on. This reflection and clarification is not for the benefit of the coach or mentor.

Use phrases such as 'This is how that came across for me', or 'This is the impact of your words on me' or even just 'Did you see what you did there?' Those are your reactions – they are your truth – and when you relay them in specific detail, you aren't judging or rating or fixing; you're simply reflecting them back in the form of an offer. When sharing observations, intuition, comments, thoughts or feelings, the coach clearly communicates that they are an 'offer' for the client to respond in any way he/she chooses.

The coach may combine the reflection with a question, in which case, we recommend that the reflection and the question are clearly separate. In this way, the coachee can hear what's being reflected back to them, and make meaning from the question, without being overwhelmed.

Here are some examples of combining a reflection with a question:

- 'You said "x". What does "x" mean for you?'
- 'You said "x" with some force just then; what's that about?'
- 'When you said "x", you shook your head. What are you feeling right now?'

But of course, the coach may just reflect back the word 'x' on its' own, for the coachee to hear, and see where that takes the conversation.

Please note that, in the Forton model, reflection is not analysing or even paraphrasing. We encourage the coach to use the coachees' own words, to reflect back a turn of phrase or a tone of voice, and not to introduce the coachs' perspective or 'translation' of 'what the coachee really meant'. This is subtly different from offering a piece of information to clarify a point. But, using the notion of 'accept, blend, and create', a reflection is an offer – for the coachee to accept or reject – as they see fit.

The Skills of Supporting

Coaching is, itself, a supportive conversation. There are, however, specific skills the coach or mentor can introduce, to reach out with specific supportive gestures. They are ways that the coach and mentor can offer a direct contribution; seed creative ideas, offer a model or paradigm; briefly teach or summarise a concept.

The coach or mentor can offer celebration for a success, encouragement as someone steps out to do something new, normalise people's fears, and enthusiasm for innovative ideas.

The supporting skill is deliberately light, concise, brief, and in support of the coachee or mentee's own knowledge and experience.

Story telling – like using a situation from one's own experience, offered as a possible example to the mentee – can then form the basis of a question – 'how might this relate to your situation?' – for example.

- 'I've seen a lot of changes in the profession, particularly in technologies, like 3D printing being brought into the surgery. How might you keep up to date with new ideas and rapid change?'
- 'I heard about a similar experience when the manager took everyone away from the workplace to have an open debate. What might be useful for you to adapt to take away from that example?'

By applying the principles of coaching, the coach is a champion for the coachee. The supporting skill is a way to demonstrate that support.

The supporting skill is also about showing support for the coaching journey itself. Coaching may sound like a natural conversation but there's a lot of focus and reflective work that goes into it; it's demanding of the coachee. Showing support for the work the coachee puts into their learning and growth is part of the role of the coach and it takes skill to avoid the obvious, or to praise the action or context alone, rather than the underlying quality.

For example, working late to get a job done may be praiseworthy occasionally, but overuse is not healthy for the coachees' work/life balance. A coach might support or encourage the *commitment* it takes to see the job through to the end, yet challenge working late on a regular basis.

Coaching is about encouraging qualities such as courage, commitment, willingness to be flexible and so on – because these qualities are transferable and will benefit other situations.

The Steps of the Coaching Conversation

Coaching and mentoring conversations have a number of steps going on in parallel: the steps in a coaching programme (for example, a series of six sessions over five months) working towards personal, professional, and career goals. Then there's the steps in the conversation itself.

The notion of 'steps' is a metaphor, an analogy for people new to coaching to have a process framework so that they can take one step after another. Another way of looking at the process is as a series of loops – the planets and orbits metaphor – accept the coach can loop backwards and forwards in the process, always in service of the coachee's learning and growth.

Purpose: Setting and Meeting Objectives

While the mentoring or coaching programme will have overall objectives, individual conversations will have their own objectives, or goals, and each of these has a purpose:

- A vision – what it will look like? (This doesn't need to be grand: you can have a vision for a perfect cup of tea; the perfect surgery layout; the best way to organise a coaching programme.)
- Values – what's important about this topic or goal?
- The ideal self – who does the mentee or coachee need to be (or become) in order to live in the new world they're creating?

It's important to accept that, in order to create a new possibility, something about the coachee also needs to change, be new, or different (ideal self). The good news is that what remains a constant are our values – those personal, social, and cultural mores that guide our behaviours in the face of change.

This is the higher level of purpose in a coaching conversation: what the coachee really wants, what matters to them about the chosen topic. At a lower level is the coaching process itself and the goal or purpose of the conversation.

Scoping Questions: The Coaching Conversation Purpose

To support the definition of conversation objectives, the mentor asks scoping questions where the mentee decides the direction of the conversation. They shouldn't be seen as placing boundaries or restrictions on the scope – if the conversation takes a new direction during the conversation which is helpful to the mentee, that is fine too. However, they can help the mentor steer away from blind alleys. The sort of questions that fit here are: What is most urgent right now? What will success look like? What is your goal? What's important about this goal – for you? What do you want to have at the end of today's session?

The vision for the future outcome is one full of all the resources the coachee needs for the vision to become reality. It's a place of partnership, where possibility, resources, and optimism come together.

Scoping the brief for a coaching session is just the start; since the ICF competences want the coach to continue in the direction of the initial stated purpose, unless the coachee indicates otherwise, then checking in at points of potential divergence is important. Asking the coachee which route they want to proceed along is the best way; this then signposts the future direction of the conversation. This is part of the partnership principle in action.

'You mentioned changing the working practises and also hiring new staff. Which is most important to look at first?'

What is the best thing that could happen? Let's think together – what is possible?

These questions frame the session and set it in its context.

At the end of the conversation some wrapping up needs to happen: as well as ensuring that the coachee summarises any insights, learning, and actions from the conversation ('takeaways'), plus any accountability steps to themselves, the coachee may need to reflect on a thorny issue; practise a new behaviour; or set themselves a challenge.

Scoping (at the start of the conversation), signposting, and wrapping up the conversation are part of the process, or structure of the coaching conversation. The coachee is responsible for the content, while the coach partners with the coachee to guide the process or structure.

It's also worth emphasising that, in the Forton model of coaching, the structure is like an exo-skeleton, visible to the coachee. Methods and tools are explained; not only describing the process of the tool, but why it's being offered. This helps the coachee understand the reason you are suggesting a particular approach, as well as giving the coachee choice in what happens in the session. This all supports the partnering principle.

One question we get asked regularly, is when is the right time for the coachee to talk about the current, undesirable state? Do we interrupt them when they go on about what they don't want? Do we let them talk themselves into a downward spiral?

Alternatively, do we ignore their need to talk about the current situation and push them into creating a vision of the desired success state?

Clearly the answer is: it depends. Sometimes people just need to vent their exasperation; they just need to be listened to for a moment. They may not be ready to 'create a vision of success'.

Whilst it's worth being aware that the feeling of being 'stuck' in old patterns may be an indication of a need for a different type of intervention (such as counselling), sometimes it's worth giving the coachee a fixed amount of time to talk through the challenge and then checking in as to whether they feel ready to shift their focus onto their goal and vision for success.

Current Reality

Once the focus for the conversation has been agreed, the future vision or desired outcome, as expressed, comes up against current realities. This is a great place for acknowledgement if today's reality is tough. It's a great place for enthusiasm from the coach if the coachee is well on the way to their goal. It's also a moment to celebrate if some success has been achieved, because this will help springboard the future success too.

The reality step is also the place to uncover the current, available resources, and it's worth really getting into detail. People so often believe that if only they had more time, money, or people, they'd succeed. The reality is, we already have so much that we overlook.

For a mentor, the reality step may be the place for a more serious conversation. If something doesn't change, there will be consequences. Here we use the 'red door/green door' metaphor:

- If you want to boost or continue your career in this direction, these things need to change such that you go through the green door. How much are you committed to this effort?
- There is an option: to find another path, career, or role. If your heart is not in your current journey, you do have the option of the red door. Would that be worth exploring before we go further?

It's worth remembering that some coachees bring other peoples' agendas to the coaching programme. Their managers' priorities; their parents' wishes; their partners' and so on. These may be valid perspectives, but the coach is there to work with the person in front of them, not these other people.

Let me give an example:

Recently I worked with someone who's manager had told them they needed to 'have a vision' for the team and what it's there to achieve within the overall purpose of the organisation. We spent time exploring what this meant, what the perspective of the manager was (through the eyes of the coachee) and it felt like the conversation was going around in circles. Then the coachee said 'I want to tell you what I really want, but I'm afraid it's going to sound stupid'. What tumbled out was a clear five-year vision for a new career direction, a 6-month plan and a 12-month goal. They were clear about the impact they wanted in the world, and how they would go about making it a reality.

It takes rapport, empathy, and a non-judgemental approach to evoke this kind of expression in a coachee and yet, once the coachee is clear about what they really want to achieve, they unlock drive, energy, and motivation towards their goal.

Tapping into the Coachees' Resourcefulness

Have you ever planned a holiday and bought new sunscreen, without first checking whether there's some in the cupboard, still in date?

In the same way, in organisations, we tend to think we need more people, money, or time, when actually we need to get smarter at using what we've already got.

The Forton model uses the acronym 'PIES' – pies feed and nourish us, just as resources – and the attitude of resourcefulness – nourish us.

PIES stands for:

- **Physical resources**
- **Intellectual resources**
- **Emotional resources**
- **Social resources.**

Resources can be within us, or in others around us. I don't need to be the expert in how to work the 3D printer, if a member of the team knows how to get the best from it. The printer is a resource, as much as the person who can work it; the person who maintains it, and the user manual, which helps us get the best from the printer.

The type of questions at this stage creates a reality check, maybe even feel limiting, because yes, there may be a gap between the desired outcome and the current state.

But this is where the coach's or mentor's questions begin to broaden out the horizon for the mentee. Questions that can help this process are:

- What have you already got (physically, intellectually, emotionally, socially)?
- On a scale of 1–10, where 10 is the desired state, where are you now?

This creates a clear picture of the gap between where the mentee is now, and where they want to be. The checklist of factors that need addressing often becomes crystal clear because of this comparison between the desired future state and the current reality.

They won't need to waste time buying more sunscreen if they've got it in the cupboard, but what about the lack of buckets and spades? Maybe that's the priority!

At this point the coach or mentor might ask: How do you feel about this now? What is your understanding of the situation? Reflecting on the situation, what is possible now?

By appreciating how much they already have, the mentee/coachee becomes more motivated to close the gap between reality and their vision – they see how much they already have. Resourcefulness is another of those 'double loop' learning qualities; once we've discovered resources in one situation, we can apply that to others.

From a motivational point of view, if the progress towards the desired vision or goal is low (say 0–4), then focusing on every possible resource will help them 'fill their boots' for the journey ahead.

One coaching client was new to an organisation, and was given a challenging task to establish an employee engagement programme, with few resources at her disposal. Her 'where are you now?' score was low, so we started with the very basics of resources;

- What have you got? (Physical) An office. A phone. Access to a photocopier. A computer.
- What's your experience to date? (Intellectual) I've done this before. I know I've got the support of the Board.
- What qualities do you have? (Emotional) I'm determined. I'm friendly and approachable. I'm organised.
- Who do you know here? (Social) There's a staff network; they have noticeboards; I can put up posters. . ..

In this way a system for consulting staff and improving employee engagement was born.

In contrast, if the 'where are you now?' score is high (7–9) it's great to focus on the goal: not just on the experience gained in the journey so far (an intellectual resource), but on how people will feel when they reach the finishing line; how they will celebrate (emotional resources); how the team will transition into the new situation (social) and so on.

New Insights – The Plan Step

At this stage, insights – or the 'aha' moments start to emerge. The mentor can begin to support the mentee in getting to grips with what's really important. At this point, the mentor may be able to suggest new ways of approaching a situation. The coach might ask questions about what the coachee might do or seed a discussion about options.

Questions that can work here are: What is one approach? What's another?

In coaching we talk about the 'mighty might': 'what *might* you do?' as distinct from decision making, 'given these factors, what *will* you do?' Exploring the mighty might gives the coachee freedom to explore different approaches, weigh up pros and cons, without risk.

Tactics

This begins the planning stage, again the mentor can offer some fresh insights, perhaps because they have dealt with similar situations. Useful questions would be:

Who do you need to involve? What resources do you need? What will you do? What is your target deadline? How will you measure success?

Overcome Barriers

The conversation then takes planning further to foresee difficulties and work through how they could be approached and overcome.

The following questions can be used: What might prevent you from succeeding? Who do you need to involve? What is missing? What can you build into the plan to avoid that from happening?

A mentor may be able to offer some useful contacts or strategies at this stage.

A coach might ask questions like: Who do you know? (social resources) who might support you? How might you find out, overcome this barrier, address this risk?

Review Steps

The planning step ends with a firm statement from the mentee or coachee summarising what they will do; by when; and how they will hold themselves accountable. They may already be accountable to a line manager or similar, but it's also important they take responsibility for their own decisions, and hold themselves to account.

Useful questions here are: What support do you need? How will you hold yourself accountable? How will you know you have been successful?

At this stage in the conversation actions are being firmed up. The mentor will be seeking commitment from the mentee to say what they are going to do and to place time and action milestones.

It's important to emphasise that it's the coachee, or mentee, who sums up here, not the Coach. This shifts ownership for the actions firmly into the coachees' lap.

For those of you running a dental practice and dealing with missed appointments, the accountability tool is a great way to help your patients or their carers be accountable for their next appointment. Invite them to say the time and date out loud, and to write it down themselves. If necessary, hand them the card and a pen; invite them to repeat the details. This act of saying and writing is one way to help them remember.

When the coachee writes down their action points it's worth giving them time to write and reflect, and not rush on too quickly.

For our coachees, asking them what will help them to remember, not only the action, but the enthusiasm and commitment to complete their goal is a great coaching tool. Find a metaphor, a picture, an image, or some words are all typical ways that coachees anchor the conversation in their mind.

The Review Step: From One Conversation to Another

The above is a review of the coaching conversation. There's also another review step, that takes place at the beginning of the next session, checking in with what's been achieved; what's not happened and, most importantly, what the coachee has learned from what has, or has not happened.

This can sometimes represent a challenge for the coach. 'Success' is so often defined as delivering or doing something. 'Failure' as not doing. And yet, in today's world, 'delegating' is not doing and yet is a highly successful way to manage time. Discovering that something didn't need to be done is also a success.

This makes it important for the coach to stay neutral and non-judgemental, when asking about 'what's happened?' 'what did you learn from what did or didn't happen?' Is another useful and non-judgemental question.

The review step at the beginning of the conversation, is a way to re-establish rapport and check in with the coachee. It should not be assumed that anything that's happened since the last time you spoke will automatically become the topic for this session's coaching. It's important to keep the review brief and then re-establish the goal, topic, or direction for today's conversation.

Reflective Learning in Coaching

The review steps in coaching are a form of reflective learning that promotes self-awareness. It also has other practical uses:

- Team Reflection: it's a method that enables a group or team to reflect together in safe spaces and non-judgemental ways.
- Ethics in Reflection: when we assume that every situation brought to the coaching/mentoring conversation has an ethical dimension, we can identify the core of the ethical issue and its relevance to technical and professional development.
- Reflection in Poor Performance: where poor performance is identified, finding the best way of giving feedback can build upon reflective practise.
- Critical reflection – supervision, mentoring, and so on

The Forton Feedback model is based upon reflective learning and can be used individually, or in groups and teams (Figure 4.3).

Typical questions you can ask in the review step, or indeed in any performance, project or programme review conversation are:

- What worked (and made a difference)?
- What do (you/I/we) need to do more of?

Figure 4.3 The feedback loop.
Student Guide, The Forton
Group, 2005.

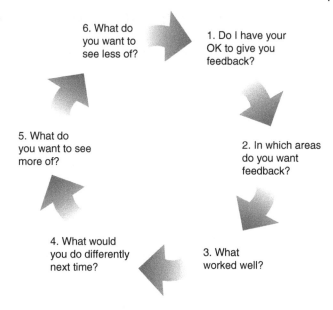

6. What do
you want to
see less of?

1. Do I have your
OK to give you
feedback?

5. What do
you want to see
more of?

2. In which areas
do you want
feedback?

4. What would
you do differently
next time?

3. What
worked well?

- What do we need to do less of?
- What do we need to stop doing?

Receiving Feedback

Of course, the other side of feedback is that of receiving it, which we all need to do from time to time.

If it helps to think of feedback as a gift, then giving, and receiving it are equally important. When we give something, it's really an 'offer' – we're not forcing things on others. The same way with feedback: if the tone is one of offering, not telling, it's left to the receiver to decide what to do with that information.

Receiving a gift takes grace and gratitude. Even if you loathe the hideous vase your mother gave you (because you happened to comment politely about it) good manners tell us to say 'thank you'. If it lives in the guest room, only to be seen on occasions, so be it.

Another way of looking at feedback is the concept of the 'high priority interrupt', which is a term from computing – it's something worth stopping and interrupting the flow for – in service of the coachee.

Negotiating how a mentor or coach might interrupt the coachee or give direct feedback to a coachee/mentee can be handled in the agreement, or contracting, stage of the relationship.

This takes us back to the early part of the coaching conversation when someone wants to talk about how bad things are: negotiating and exploring with the coachee as to how you might interrupt them, in service of them achieving their goals.

Assuming that feedback will happen, and that reflective practice is expected, will start the working relationship on a sound footing. Ask them 'How would you like to receive feedback during the coaching session?' rather than 'Would you like feedback?'

The 'Field', or the World of the Coachee

Put simply, our world is made up of the resources we have; those we don't have yet available to us; the location of those resources; the means of accessing those resources; and the gateways to, and barriers to, those resources.

In the Forton model we call these:

- Resources – 'PIES' (already referred to above)
- Domains – the location of resources (internal, external, individual, groups)
- Structures – the visible and invisible gateways and barriers that allow us to access, or deny us access to, resources

A physical resource – this book, for example – contains information (intellectual) which may interest the reader (emotional), who may share it as a useful resource with others (social).

The book resides in the domain of the library, bookshop or warehouse (external, group).

You can access this book by paying for it, or by going to a library to take it out on loan. For the former you need the resource of money; for the latter, some form of permission (library card). If your credit is good, or your library card up to date, you have access. If not, access is denied to you.

To achieve access, you may need to use influencing skills to convince someone and you'll need to have the intellectual capacity to know who to approach and how to go about this.

To most people, getting hold of a book is an unconscious process, one way or another. It's no different when we think about the resources we are trying to unlock every day at work.

- Who's in charge of ordering the personal protective equipment (PPE)?
- Who's making the decision about new equipment?
- How do I put my case for a new waiting room system?

Talking it through can help break down the process towards resources – and stops us assuming that 'more time, people, and money' are the only resource solutions, to which many leaders and managers default, unless they have the time to talk it through with a coach or mentor.

There are less tangible resources – we might also have access to enthusiasm, an emotional resource, or to our intuition, an intellectual resource.

When coachees explore the Field, they unlock the secrets to their systems: who to approach; what's needed to get the goal I'm looking to achieve; when's the best time to put this proposal to the practice principal?

When people identify resources and see the field of play clearly, it gives them greater confidence to move forward.

References

Cambridge Dictionary (2020) definition of skill; https://dictionary.cambridge.org/dictionary/english, accessed 21 May 2020.

Collins Dictionary (2020) definition of skill; https://www.collinsdictionary.com/dictionary/english, accessed 21 May 2020.

Covey, S.M.R. (2006). *The Speed of Trust: The One Thing that Changes Everything*. Fraanklin Covey.

International Coach Federation, (2021). Coaching Competences: https://coachfederation.org/core-competencies.

International Coach Federation (ICF), assessment markers, https://coachfederation.org/pcc-markers, accessed 21 May 2020.

Forton Professional Leadership Coaching Training Programme Student Guide, Lindsay J., The Forton Group 2005.

Scottish Qualifications Authority (2008). *The Routledge International Encyclopedia of Education* (eds. G. McCulloch and D. Crook). Routledge https://www.sqa.org.uk/sqa/83655.html (accessed 5 November 2020).

5

Practical Case Studies

The purpose of this book is to drive practical change and the case studies in this chapter form its main focus. We have included a range of projects developed by dental professionals and used in the real world of dentistry and all of these projects are practitioner-focused, rather than academic. Contributors were invited to provide an overview of their project through an online survey and the authors are very grateful for their generous participation.

Background to the Case Studies

Improving UK Dental Service Quality

The Regulation of Dental Services Programme Board (RDSPB) was established in England in 2014 to look at streamlining regulation of the dental profession, with the aim of improving the quality of care received by patients. Membership of the Board includes the Care Quality Commission (CQC), the Department of Health and Social Care (DHSC), the General Dental Council (GDC), and NHS England (NHSE). The work of the Board is supported and underpinned by, the NHS Business Services Authority, (NHSBSA), Healthwatch England (HWE) and the local Healthwatch network.

The RDSPB's key areas of focus were to define a system of quality improvement in the dental sector and the role of key stakeholders in improvement.

The model below (Figure 5.1) illustrates the four stages of performance concern from no concern to severe concern, and recognises that earlier intervention and remedial action can reverse the flow. For example, formal supervision can prevent a moderate concern progressing to a severe concern. If concerns arise, a proportionate structured approach would be used, involving peer support, followed by more direct supervision and finally externally governed sanctions. This concept has been shared with key national stakeholders and local professional dental network members and it has received significant support.

The Board is now looking to the profession to participate in the self-help process, to consider time for peer review. For example, for Local Dental Networks (LDNs) and Local Dental Committees (LDCs) to help re-energise local peer review and PASS services and shift the balance of regulation closer to local resolution and prevention.

Practical Applications of Coaching and Mentoring in Dentistry, First Edition.
Janine Brooks and Helen Caton-Hughes.

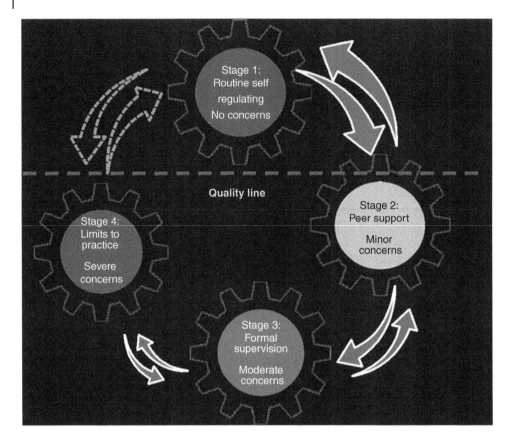

Figure 5.1 RDSPB quality improvement framework. *Source:* RDSPB, A model for quality improvement across the dental sector, 2017.

Underpinning Concepts

It is recognised that only a small proportion of all practitioners and practices are of concern and that the framework is as much about maintaining good practice as it is about preventing poor practice from emerging.

The framework encourages an open learning culture, with structured peer support between professionals, where dental clinicians primarily monitor and regulate their own clinical performance.

The RDSPB published a report in December 2015 looking at the future of dental service regulation. It included areas of quality or performance and this is taken from that section:

> Where issues of quality or performance are identified, there is limited and inconsistent support available to help dentists to improve services. By this, we mean there is little support for 'failing' practices/vulnerable practitioners and in the general context of quality improvement more widely across the dental sector.

It seems reasonable to suggest that the support that RDSPB have identified as limited or inconsistent could be provided by trained mentors.

In 2017 the GDC consultation paper 'Shifting the Balance' (2017) also advocated moving the emphasis for addressing performance concerns closer to local resolution and prevention.

> The GDC wants to work with the profession and our partners to build on the good practice that already exists to maximise the potential of local resolution.

Postgraduate Medical and Dental Education (PGMDE) (previously known as Deaneries) are now part of local HEE teams and have an important role to play in providing support at a local level.

The Role of Coaching and Mentoring in Supporting Dental Service Quality

> Activities such as coaching and mentoring, where individuals are supported by other members of the dental profession, also have an important role to play here, and are valuable ways of enhancing the skills and approach of all involved.
>
> *(Shifting the balance, GDC)*

The benefits of working with a mentor cannot be underestimated in helping professionals keep on the right track. A mentor can assist their mentee to deepen reflective thinking and extract maximum learning from CPD activities for the benefit of patients. Importantly a well-trained mentor can support an individual to ensure their learning is translated into improved ways of working and direct improvements to patient care. This underpins the assurance that improvements are fully embedded within the professional's daily practice.

By linking local and national processes concerned with performance and development of dental professionals, resources can be more effectively utilised and ultimately support better patient care.

When considering underperformance of a practitioner there are many factors that can contribute, for example:

- Mental health issues
- Drug/alcohol abuse
- Breakdown of family relationships
- Overwork
- Physical illness
- Poor skills in clinical care
- Poor organisation and managerial skills in the delivery of health care
- Knowledge, skills, and attitudes that are below accepted standards
- A lack of clinical competence
- Behaviour problems.

In addition, there are more regular indicators of performance issues, such as a high number of complaints.

The Case Study Projects

The questions asked of each project lead included a project description, outline, and category, plus a summary of the practical messages arising from the project and their potential (or actual) wider relevance.

Case Study Categories

We identified five categories, which are described below.

1) Dentists in Difficulty including PASS
2) Evaluation
3) Early years – Undergraduates, Foundation dentists, and post foundation
4) General Practice and organisational culture
5) Models/Tools.

Category One Case Studies: Dentists in Difficulty Including PASS

The first group of projects are those that demonstrate practical applications of mentoring to locally support colleagues who are struggling and having difficulty.

These projects have been designed to help and support dentists who are struggling, mainly with issues of performance. They are aligned to organisations which underpin the work and all projects work within those structures.

Local Dental Committee (LDC)

LDC's in the UK were set up in 1948, at the inception of the NHS. There are a total of 110 LDCs across the UK. LDC's are not recognised in statute in all areas of the UK. Scotland and Northern Ireland differ from England and Wales in terms of 'official' representation.

Where LDC's are recognised in statute they represent dentists who are on the NHS Performers List in the locality covered geographically by the LDC. However, many LDC's represent dentists who work in Community Dental Services (CDS) and other sectors of dental practice where this has been agreed locally. The body of the LDC consists of NHS general dental practitioners (GDP's) along with secondary care and community service representatives. Many LDC's have set up PASS services (see below) for their local area although this is not universal across the UK and schemes operate differently from area to area.

Practitioner Advice and Support Scheme (PASS)

The first PASS was established in East Lancashire in 1999 The concept of PASS was introduced to help those dentists who for one reason or another were in need of additional support. It was first designed for those dentists in difficulty to be supported or mentored by experienced colleagues within the same region where they worked, and the intention has remained broadly the same.

PASS Aims and Objectives

The ambition of a PASS is to be able to support the dentist in difficulty such that they can continue in practice with their confidence restored and able to further contribute in an effective way within the profession.

The overall aim of a PASS is to provide skilled mentoring support including advice and guidance to dentists who are struggling with issues impacting on their ability to perform to required standards for dental practitioners. This may include a particular area of practice; following a patient complaint or a practice management concern.

The purpose of PASS is to provide support at an early stage before performance concerns arise or escalate, by providing dentists with skilled support and guidance to help them improve their performance.

PASS Processes

In most situations PASS is coordinated and facilitated by LDC's and over the past few years PASS has become an important additional tool in the efforts to address the complaints or performance issues that colleagues face.

Dentists in need of support may self-refer to the PASS coordinator or, more commonly, be referred to the scheme by the NHSE Area Team Performance Advisory Group (PAG). When a colleague has entered the process they are initially assessed and then passed to a member of the PASS team for the most appropriate support. This may simply be signposting but might involve a series of one to one mentoring meetings or perhaps onward referral to HEE or health support.

Funding streams will vary from one scheme to another but there may well be an initial contribution towards the costs from the LDC with further costs being met by the mentee.

Case Study One

Thames Valley PASS
Contributor: Dr. Barkat Ahmed BDS

This project is designed to help GDPs in the region who may have encountered difficulties in their working lives. It is for dentists who have been 'flagged up' but it also allows self-referral and access for GDPs who are having concerns but are not necessarily having problems with regulations, etc.

There will be an opportunity for potential mentees to seek a mentor who can help them in their development, without them being concerned about specific issues. This approach would allow a pro-active and preventative approach, which will serve all stakeholders much better.

Programme Success Indicators

The programme has several indicators for success. These are to –

- Provide a point of referral for anyone concerned about a dentist
- Identify the appropriate level of intervention
- Provide support for dentists in difficulty through intervention at an appropriate stage
- Support dentists where necessary

- Provide appropriately skilled members able to assist the professional
- Audit activity.

The PASS group has a committee, which meets on an ad-hoc basis and is constituted of –

- Two LDC representatives, nominated by each of the three LDCs in the Thames Valley (total of six LDC representatives)
- One Dental Practice Adviser from NHSE
- One Consultant in Dental Public Health
- One lay representative
- One HEE representative
- One NHSE team commissioner
- One Local Professional Network (LPN) member (co-opted).

The group adheres to Nolan Principles, Committee on Standards in Public Life, (1995). These are seven principles of behaviour and culture which those in public service are expected to demonstrate.

It is planned to increase the LDC representatives to three with an emphasis on younger members.

From the above group a chair, secretary, and treasurer is selected. Committee members take on other roles, for example; electronic communication and engagement (mainly through social media channels as well as the traditional methods). Each role is held on a three-year basis, with elections held if needed. Each person nominated also needs to be seconded. There is a deadline each year in June for recruiting new members. The PASS group recruits dentists to the Committee from the local area, and advertises via social media. Further promotion is through the LDC, British Dental Association (BDA), and other study groups.

In addition, people with a non-dental background from local groups that already have some affiliation with healthcare or mentoring can be recruited. It is the role of the secretary to receive the applications for potential new members. The telephone contacts of the secretary and chairman are available should a potential member wish to call and discuss anything before applying. This makes it easier for potential mentors to have their queries answered before joining.

Potential members will have a questionnaire to complete in terms of what suitability they feel that they have for their role and the potential skills that they can bring. It is important to have a programme of recruitment and selection of mentors, as well as the mentees. All mentors need to be trained appropriately and the learning needs of the mentors are identified through learning surveys and interviews.

A combination of assessment methods has been shown to be most effective, rather than a single method. The project recruits mentors that have been trained via a variety of programmes that are validated for example by the Institute of Leadership and Management (ILM), as well other leading organisations such as the European Mentoring and Coaching Council (EMCC). In addition, mentoring courses such as the four-day Oxford Deanery programme can be a good place for recruiting new mentors.

It is important that the recruitment process, as well as the expectations and criteria are fully explained to the mentors. This needs to be explained early on, especially the amount of time they are expected to invest, as this is often the most precious resource for the mentor. The mentors should also have continuous support. They should get frequent and constructive feedback from their cases and this should assist in their goal setting. The feedback can be given orally, as well as written. All mentors should have an annual evaluation and any support needed should be provided. Ideally once there are more mentors, those that are more experienced can do case reviews and reflections with the junior ones.

Referrals to the Mentoring Scheme

It is important for a potential referral to have as many routes into the programme as possible. All members of the committee can receive referrals through email, phone or other social media contact. There is an online presence through the website and electronic communication gives a point of contact. Anyone who has a concern or a potential concern about a dentist's performance can make a referral. The main routes are via dental care professionals (DCPs), LDC members, the Local Area Team (LAT) via the Performers List Decision Panel (PLDP) or PAG, and of course self-referrals.

Initial contacts are passed to the secretary who convenes a decision group. The decision group assesses whether the referral is appropriate. A minimum of three members discuss the best course of action. Once the decision group has decided that the case is an appropriate case, a lead is appointed from the membership group. The committee aims to distribute cases evenly so as not to over-burden any particular mentor. The lead contacts the referred practitioner for an initial face-to-face meeting. This can be an e-meet through Skype or any other appropriate software. Research has shown this to be effective compared to face-to-face meetings. It is important to try and do this as soon as possible but the aim is within three days. The case lead will be responsible for working with the practitioner to identify the support required, facilitating the support and providing feedback to the Decisions group. The case lead will not necessarily directly provide the support as there may be somebody more appropriate in the committee or an external referral may be required. If the case is felt to be suitable for the committee, then the mentee will be given the name of their mentor in writing.

Ideally the mentee should have a choice of mentor but this may be affected by the appropriateness of the training that the mentor has. The mentor should than contact the mentee. The first meeting with the practitioner is anticipated to take about 60–90 minutes, the aim of which is to formulate an action plan with SMART objectives. The case lead will then provide the practitioner with a written copy of the action plan within five days. All records are kept in accordance with the Data Protection Act 1998 and periodic audits are carried out.

Initially three triple hour sessions are provided. These are in the form of coaching and mentoring, where the aim is for the practitioner to gain insight and to develop, as well as appreciate the current resources that they have, and construct an agreement explaining each person's responsibilities and so that boundaries are set. The mentee is given a chance to input into what they agree to as the boundaries and their consent confirmed.

If the mentee is not forthcoming a reminder letter should be written 10 days after the initial meeting. Should there be no contact after that the case is referred back to the decision group, who can decide on the next appropriate step, which will be one of the following:

- No further action is required.
- The case raises some cause for concern and the practitioner could benefit from support from a PASS member/mentor.
- The issues raised by the case would be better addressed by another agency, e.g. NHSE contracts team, Dentists' Health Support Programme (DHSP), and HEE Thames Valley.

- The issues discovered should be dealt with under the NHS Complaints Scheme.
- The allegations/issues are of such gravity that the case should be referred back to the originator with advice to contact another body, e.g. the GDC, NHSE performance lead.
- The practitioner be formally supported by the HEE Thames Valley and Wessex (TV&W) coach/mentor programme.

There is the possibility that there may be some issues that are not appropriate for the mentoring group to deal with alone. For example:

- Contract management issues, where there are no other aspects of poor performance.
- Education and training issues.
- Alcohol and substance abuse issues.
- Where health issues are the main reason for the poor performance.
- Suspected fraud or criminal activity.
- Poor performance that has already caused harm (physical, mental or financial) to patients/staff/public.
- Foundation dentists, where the Deanery should be the first point of contact.
- Those already receiving support from elsewhere, e.g. Postgraduate Deanery.

It should be noted that there might still be some involvement required of the group and this should be taken as a positive as it will allow greater visibility and be able to achieve a successful outcome.

In rolling out and implementation of the mentoring programme, the following points were noted as being of importance:

- Programme co-ordination, teamwork is facilitated, there is seen to be respect, accountability, and trust, as well as evaluation of the programme.
- Sufficient human resources present from the outset.
- Contribution from committee members, it cannot be left to one or two individuals to take on the burden of operating the programme.
- Resources are secured. There should be funding from the LAT – the benefits of the programme highlighted to them as well as from HEE. The LDC should also fund the programme – although this will raise the potentially-problematic issue of NHS practitioners funding being used for non-NHS dentists.
- Multiple sources are used to identify the individual's needs. These will help to improve the quality of the training; they will be in the form of a formal questionnaire, as well as informal networking and meetings.
- Effective communication between and among the programme participants. This will be done in addition to the committee meetings so that there is ongoing contact, rather than the quarterly formal meetings.

It is also important to celebrate successes and recognise achievements regularly, as these will enhance the reputation of the programme and increase its' visibility. It is anticipated that the local BDA, and other dental and non-dental organisations will be contacted. The success of all mentoring programmes depends on having engaged and fulfilled expectations for all participants: mentors, mentor trainers, mentees, and project leaders.

Word of mouth is still the best way to pass on information to advise potential mentors, as well as any mentees who may be looking for support. It has far reaching consequences, affective/emotional, cognitive, and behavioural for all participants, as well as the wider community. Another way to raise awareness is to network. This will be done by seeking out other mentoring programmes, which are already working. This will allow building wider relationships outside of the geographical boundaries and as such sharing and developing ideas that will benefit the programme.

Mentoring Group Evaluation

Once having set up the mentoring group it is important to be able to evaluate it. Evaluation of the programme will help to look for any necessary adjustments needed, and thus have an impact on the effectiveness of the programme. Evaluation can be summative – collected on completion of the programme to see if it has been effective, or formative – collected during the programme to help improve it. Research has shown that a combination of the two types is most effective. However, as the programme is starting out, it will be more heavily focused on formative evaluation information. Once it has been established, much more emphasis on summative evaluation can be placed. As part of this, there needs to be consideration as to what kind of information would be most useful. It is important to get the perspective of both the mentors and the mentees.

- For mentors, we need to assess if they feel well supported; can achieve their goals and have developmental plans in place.
- For the mentees, it is important that they can see how the programme will help them and how, by using the programme their perception of themselves in their professional role has been affected.

To collect meaningful information and assess its impact, it is crucial to have descriptive data: including ethnic group, gender, age, and years of experience.

In evaluating quality, it is important to assess the programme process outcomes, which are all set at a target of 100%. The three objectives measured are that:

1) All mentees will have SMART goals following their meeting with the case lead.
2) There will be at least three meetings in the first year.
3) At the end of these meetings a developmental plan will be established, which may include having further meetings.

It is also important to evaluate the participant experience and their perceptions, these will be to assess the value perceived by the programme participants, the mutual trust level and appropriateness of the match.

Lastly, the programme as a whole needs to be evaluated, as well as the effect that it has had. This is assessed by the overall satisfaction felt by participants, as well as the rating of the administration and support received. An annual report will be published on the website of the PASS scheme.

Practical messages:

- Support and advice group run by dentists for dentists.
- 'You are not alone'. To let all those who need it know that there are others going through the same as them and that there are people to share and support them.
- 'Prevention is better than cure'.

Table 5.1 Thames Valley PASS – lessons learned.

Lessons	Changes made (after lesson learned)
Not able to recognise those who need it. 'Surprised' by those who have asked about it.	Kept my approach 'open'. Try not to have bias, (not easily done).
Has to be inclusive to all, we are all part of the same family.	None major, but reiterated to keep in mind belief.
Has to be focused on prevention rather than intervention approach.	Try to allow earlier access.

Wider relevance of the case study:

There are currently high levels of stress and dissatisfaction amongst those working in the profession and the long term aspects of this should be considered, as ultimately this will lead to diminished patient care. Mentoring can minimise stress and dissatisfaction by:

- Acknowledging that dentistry is a highly stressful profession and dental professionals are not expected to be continuously functioning, as if they were a machine.
- Knowing it is good to talk and share concerns.
- Working together to support each other.

Case Study Two

The Dorset PASS
Contributor: Mrs. Sarah Jackson BDS

This voluntary scheme has been running for over 10 years. A group of seven facilitate the scheme and are comprised of three members of the LDC, two post graduate tutors from Dorchester and Bournemouth, the Dental Practice Adviser, and a lay person.

Scheme Aims
- Protect patients through early detection of under performance by dentists
- Support dentists by providing them with skilled support and guidance to help them improve their performance and cope with problems they may be having
- Provide a point of referral for the profession, The Wessex Area Team, and other concerned bodies
- Assure the public, politicians, and the profession that the issue of performance is being addressed responsibly

Definitions
The scheme describes under performance by a dental professional as:

- Actions that place patients at risk
- Failure to meet accepted and required standards
- Departure from what is considered normal practice

Process

Whilst participation in the scheme is voluntary, if a dentist declines to be involved then the case would be referred to The Wessex Area Team. The first step for a referral is a local investigation by the PASS service. If this fails to resolve the issues, then the Wessex Area Team and Practitioner Performance Advice (PPA) (formally The National Clinical Assessment Service) will be informed.

There are a number of routes into the programme, which include:

- Self-referral
- The Wessex Area Team
- Worried colleague(s) or member(s) of staff
- NHSBSA
- Routine practice inspections.

Confidentiality

Confidentiality is an important aspect of the scheme and, wherever possible, the identity of a whistle-blower is protected. Please see the note on whistleblowing at the end of the case study. The identity of the dentist under review is also kept confidential within the scheme as disclosure is on a strictly 'need to know' basis. The minimum necessary information is used and everyone party to the identity of the dentist is aware of their responsibilities. These criteria follow Caldicott guidelines (UK Caldicott Guardian Council 2017). In addition, all documentation is shredded at the end of each PASS meeting. An anonymised report is prepared for The Wessex Area Team and Dorset LDC at the year end.

Details can be found on the Dorset LDC website and the PASS leaflet or by contacting The Wessex Area Team.
Visit: http://www.dorsetldc.org.

Practical messages:
- Be confidential
- Be non-judgmental
- Have good listening skills

Wider relevance of the case study

Other dentists setting up PASS services may find it useful to see how one that is currently active works. Also it showed how we ensure that dentists are aware of the scheme, so that it is used. Specific points identified are:

- Have good communication skills
- Be a good ambassador for the profession
- Be approachable

Table 5.2 Dorset PASS – lessons learned.

Lessons	Changes made (after lesson learned)
The value of asking open questions	Be less direct
More confident in my ability to mentor dentists in difficulty	Ask more open questions
Different approaches which I could use to mentor	

Whistleblowing note

The following is taken from Freedom to speak up: 'Should any primary care employees wish to make a protected disclosure, they can do so via a prescribed organisation under the Public Interest Disclosure Order 1999' National Guardian's Office (2019). NHSE is a prescribed organisation, meaning that individuals raising concerns with NHSE are protected from detrimental treatment or victimisation from their employers after they have made a qualifying disclosure. Each prescribed organisation under the act has a remit to receive disclosures relating to a specific subject. NHSE is able to receive disclosures relating to the delivery of primary medical, dental, ophthalmic, and pharmaceutical services in England. In order to qualify for protection under the Order, any disclosure must:

1) Relate to information about malpractice (including criminal offences, failure to comply with legal obligations, miscarriages of justice, threats to health and safety of an individual, damage to the environment) and a deliberate attempt to cover up any of the above.
2) Be in the public interest (the worker must have reasonable belief that the information shows that one of the categories of wrongdoing listed in the legislation has occurred or is likely to occur).
3) Have been raised in the right way.
4) Have been made in good faith.

Other organisations with a prescribed status relating to primary dental care are:

- The CQC
- HWE
- The GDC
- HEE
- NHS Improvement (formerly Monitor and the Trust Development Authority)
- The NHSBSA
- The Secretary of State for Health.

Source: NHSE (2017, pp. 9–10). Freedom to speak up in primary care. Guidance to primary care providers on supporting whistleblowing in the NHS.

Case Study Three

Dentists in Difficulty Including PASS
Contributor: Dr. Sumair Khan BDS

Outline:

This case study was developed in response to growing concerns about dentists in difficulty. This was underpinned by a recognition that increasing numbers of GDC registrants appear to be struggling. Some of the factors that impact on practitioners were identified as:

- Regulation and legislation, for example HTM01–05; GDPR; National Institute for Clinical Excellent (NICE); CQC; constant updating of recommendations, guidance, and regulatory requirements. Many practitioners struggle to keep up to date and/or manage the target driven nature of dentistry.

- Numbers of complaints and fitness to practise hearings – many overseas qualified prac-titioners are unfamiliar with UK working environments; many performers work in isola-tion (even within larger practices). There is a feeling that patients are more demanding and litigious; some practices struggle with patient feedback and complaints. Less experi-enced graduates and foundation dentists may struggle more. There is also an increase in the numbers of registrants reporting fellow registrants (blue on blue).
- Cases reported by indemnity providers.
- The level of fees for GDC registration and for indemnity can be difficult for some practitioners.

Project aims
- Develop the capability of HEE TV&W Postgraduate Dental Team to support dentists in difficulty.
- Ensure the support for dentists in difficulty is effective and efficient and can easily meet the demand for the service.
- Ensure a high quality mentoring programme through recruitment, training, and quality assurance (QA).

Process
The project used a four-phase plan to introduce a coaching and mentoring programme to support dentists in difficulty.

1) Stakeholder engagement; evaluation of resources and capacity to deliver the service; setting objectives.
2) Recruitment and training of mentors, establishing mentoring agreements and the pro-cess to be followed.
3) Mentees recruited/identified and matched with mentors. Both parties to ensure they follow the terms of the mentoring agreements and the process. TV&W (provider of the service) support and monitor this stage carefully.
4) Collation of feedback from both mentees and mentors, and discussion of the outcomes of the programme with stakeholders. Also learning from the feedback and making appropriate changes to the agreements or the processes.

Practical messages:
- Recruiting and training coach-mentors can be time consuming.
- Establishing agreements and protocols for interactions between mentors and mentees are vital.
- Learning from the outcomes and feedback to make changes, so that the agreements and protocols can evolve and become more effective. The programme must be dynamic.

Wider relevance of the case study:
The regulatory and educational support teams within dentistry need to develop a more empathetic and supportive culture and stop concentrating on penalising, punishing, and escalating under-performance

- Mindfulness and well-being of healthcare professionals must be borne in mind at all stages.
- Developing a culture of support and empathy for those healthcare professionals who are under-performing/struggling.
- Learning from and demonstrating the value of coaching and mentoring within healthcare.

Table 5.3 Dentists in difficulty including PASS – lessons learned.

Lessons	Changes made (after lesson learned)
Mentoring is also incredibly rewarding for the mentor – not necessarily financially.	A dentist in difficulty has been recruited to be part of the HEE TV&W Dental Team of coach/mentors.
Mentoring can be stressful and mentors require support throughout the programme.	Regular review and revision of the protocols and arrangements for coach mentoring.
It is important for mentees to have continuing access to support networks after the initial process/sessions.	Regular meetings with the mentees

Case Study Four

Designing and Implementing a Mentoring Scheme in Birmingham
Contributor: Dr. Ahmad El-Toudmeri BDS

Background

The Birmingham LDC was established in 1977 and the membership is elected by Birmingham based dentists.

The impetus to the scheme came from studies that showed an unacceptable level of ill health and lack of well-being within the profession. A BDA report demonstrated that almost half of GDPs (47%) surveyed in June/July 2014 reported low levels of life satisfaction, with a similar proportion (44%) reporting low levels of happiness. In addition, around 6 out of 10 respondents reported experiencing high levels of anxiety during the day prior to being surveyed. In addition;

- Stress cited as the number one cause of sick days in the NHS.
- The suicide rate for dentists is twice as high as the general population and three times that of white collar workers.
- Coronary disease and high blood pressure are over 25% more prevalent among dentists than in the general population.

Added to the health concerns, external factors such as an increasing threat of litigation and increasing patient demands and expectation were noted to impact on an individuals' resilience.

Identified Pressures

Issues that impact on an individual dentists' ability for optimum performance include:

- **Isolation** – many dentists practice alone, so do not have the support of peers and colleagues. There can be considerable competition in dentistry. Sometimes this can be amongst peers within a practice and this can lead to problems between practitioners.
- **Confinement** – the average dentist spends most of their working day in a small surgery, sometimes without a window. The treatment of patents is intricate and performed in a small, restricted oral space. Interventions can be both physically and mentally taxing and as a result, strain, back troubles, circulatory disorders, and fatigue are common.

- **Economic** – many dentists face a number of financial demands, including mortgages, dental practice loans, indemnity fees, registration fees, income tax, and other professional and personal financial commitments.
- **Dental Contract** – systems of remuneration can be challenging, as can the threat of clawback and withdrawal of the contract. Targets can add pressure to an individual.
- **Burn out** can become an increasing issue.
- **Time Pressures** – trying to see patients on time, patients can be upset if their appointment is delayed. Trying to maintain a work/life balance.
- **Patient Pressures** – working with anxious or poorly cooperating patients can lead to stress. Meeting patient demands and high expectations can be problematic. Evidence of paralleling dentist emotions with that of patients.

Identified Solutions

A number of remedies were identified as being of help in easing or minimising these issues:

- Improve work environment.
- Improve communication with colleagues.
- Work more regular hours and taking time out for holidays/relaxation.
- Physical exercise.
- Taking up a hobby.
- MENTORING + COACHING!

It is the last of these remedies that this case study decided to use.

Scheme Aims:

- To provide dental practitioners with support, advice, and guidance in their professional and personal lives.
- To provide a 'safe place' for open, confidential, and non-judgemental advice.

A preventive or minimising approach is fostered to allow for the early identification of dental practitioners whose performance may be of concern and to provide appropriate support before serious concerns develop.

The scheme is open to dental practitioners and other members of the dental team who are Birmingham based. The LDC was responsible for setting up the scheme and provide ongoing maintenance. This includes initial and ongoing training for mentors, funding for the mentoring and an online presence through the LDC website.

Process

The scheme has four main sections. These are: the initial referral into the scheme; the linking of an individual with a mentor; the actual mentoring and finally evaluation. Following evaluation an individual may re-enter mentoring.

Routes in:

- Self-referral – if a practitioner feels that they would benefit from the support or assistance.
- A concerned colleague or member of staff.
- Referral by the LAT.

- Referral by the PAG.
- Referral by other bodies – such as the GDC.

1) Referral:

Referral of a practitioner into the programme is a confidential process. Online referral can be made via a secure proforma. Once a referral has been received there are a number of next steps:

- No action required.
- Not appropriate for intervention – alternative action is required.
- Referral accepted.

2) Linking:

Once a referral is considered to be appropriate for the programme the referred practitioner is linked to a mentor. Matching is based on clinical background, experience, and personal attributes. Mentoring is a two-way process and fruitless if both parties are unable to develop rapport.

Conflicts of interest are important and must be minimised. Dentistry on a local level is a very small world. Some mentees may not wish to know their mentors on a personal level and so it may be of benefit if one could opt to refer themselves to a PASS service further afield.

3) Mentoring:

It is important that the mentoring relationship is open and honest and the purpose is discussed at the outset. Goals are set with the mentee and it is made clear that the process is not punitive but supportive. In addition, a timetable is set and agreed between the mentor and mentee.

Possible areas have been identified which may give particular concern, these are:

- Behavioural and health issues (such as alcohol or drug abuse).
- Poor clinical standards and/or patient care.
- Poor practice management.
- Frequent complaints.
- Suspected fraudulent or criminal behaviour.

4) Evaluation:

The importance of this step cannot be understated and it should not be confused with the review step. Reviewing progress at the start of each session is an important part of the mentoring pathway, however this step refers to the evaluation process of the pathway in and of itself.

It is hoped that evaluation will be completed not only by the participating mentor but also by the mentee. Good evaluation will allow the mentoring group to reflect on what happened and what was learnt from the process which leads to greater insight and improvements and refinements to the scheme. Questionnaires are the main tool of evaluation. Follow up with the referring body is also included.

Practical messages:

- Modern dentistry is becoming ever more stressful as a result of a number of factors and cultural environment.

- PASS services are invaluable for providing dental practitioners with support, advice, and guidance in a 'safe place'.
- The mentoring journey has to flow from one step to the next to ensure quality of the process.

Wider relevance of the project

PASS services and more broadly mentoring schemes can be of great benefit to all levels of the dental profession – as it currently stands our PASS can only provide mentoring for dental practitioners – however this neglects a large part of the wider dental team. In order to provide the most effective healthcare to our patients – access to invaluable services such as PASS must be made available to all dental professionals.

- Healthcare professionals must feel that they are supported both in their personal and professional lives in order to allow them to provide the best possible healthcare to their patients.
- More work needs to be done to reduce the stigma around asking for help – healthcare professionals should not be made to worry about this being used against them.
- Those that need help the most are often those least likely to seek it – so there must be active promotion of any help that may be provided to increase awareness.

Table 5.4 Birmingham PASS – lessons learned.

Lessons	Changes made (after lesson learned)
It can be difficult to overcome preconceptions in established organisations – especially with implementing a PASS scheme.	Providing presentations and delivering information in a suitable manner for the organisation to accept and digest. In addition, allowing questions to be asked of the process and open scrutiny to all the stages – as a result the barriers that may be long established in opposition to a PASS scheme as a result of preconceptions or bad personal experience, etc. can be avoided.
There will be pressures from various organisations to change the aims or the outcomes of the process in order to benefit their agenda – often to the detriment of the mentee (e.g. regulatory bodies offering an incoming referral pathway for mentees in exchange for information or performance reports).	Staying true to the process and knowing how to stand firm to preserve the aims of the process.
Uptake of mentees in the process can be much lower than originally planned for and anticipated.	Promoting the mentoring scheme in various novel ways in order to reach those who may need it the most. In addition, ensuring to continue mentoring even when the PASS scheme may have no mentees to ensure that deskilling doesn't occur.

Category Two Case Studies-Evaluation

Evaluation is an important step to demonstrate a programme's success. It helps to understand what works, what doesn't, and why. It helps identify areas for improvement and is critical for promoting accountability. Without evaluation it is impossible to determine if the introduction of mentoring has achieved any worthwhile benefits.

Evaluation should be built into a project at the planning stage: to establish what is to be evaluated and methods of measurement. For any evaluation, the metrics selected have to be meaningful, measurable, and objective.

When considering evaluation of a mentoring project several aspects need to be included. For example:

- The process introduced
- Outcomes
- Satisfaction of the mentors and mentees
- Cost effectiveness.

Some of the case studies above have included their evaluation step. Often evaluation is undertaken at the end of a project, however wherever possible evaluation during the project can be useful in preventing the project veering off course and to allow modifications to be made at an earlier stage.

Taylor et al. (2005) defines evaluation as:

'Put simply, evaluation by members of a project or organisation will help people to learn from their day-to-day work. It can be used by a group of people, or by individuals working alone. It assesses the effectiveness of a piece of work, a project, or a programme. It can also highlight whether your project is moving steadily and successfully towards achieving what it set out to do, or whether it is moving in a different direction. You can then celebrate and build on successes as well as learn from what has not worked so well'.

Evaluation is a critical part of all the case studies within this chapter. The specific case studies in this section take evaluation as the main driver: *evaluation is* the case study, which makes them particularly interesting.

Case Study Five

An Evaluation Methodology: A Piece of Reflective Writing for PAG
Contributor: Dr. Claudia Peace BDS

Outline

This case study looks at the evaluation of reflective writing submitted to a PAG from performers for whom there is a concern. It is quite common practice when dealing with a complaint to request a reflection from the performer. Whilst it is relatively simple to recognise a good or bad piece of reflective writing there is no accepted objective way to score the writing. Such a method would help to ensure the assessment of reflective writing is consistent, transparent, and fair.

One example of an outcome could be 'how many performers are remediated?'. In analysing that question, we can ask ourselves what are the areas in which the performer has reached the required standard?; how do we know they've reached that standard? and what can we look at to assess it?

An area to assess is reflective writing. If the reflection is done well, it can be useful in demonstrating insight and remediation. However, when done badly, it lets a performer down, potentially leading to escalation to a PLDP which has much more serious consequences.

This project seeks to turn a subjective assessment into an objective, measurable exercise.

Since demonstrating insight about performance is an important part of remediation measures have been chosen that demonstrate it. These are:

1) Acknowledgement of the issue, (identification of why the issue arose).
2) The performer's responsibility identified.
3) What the performer has learned from the experience.
4) What the performer would do differently if it happened again.
5) Whether there is a training need as a consequence.
6) Where the performer can identify some useful CPD.

A maximum score of six is allocated. Six being excellent, five being very good; four good; three room for improvement; two, poor reflection: one, very poor, and 0, no reflection at all. Any performer who scores four or over will have shown a good piece of reflective writing.

Applying the criteria makes it easier to evaluate the reflection in an objective manner. In addition, the evaluation of the reflection assists in helping to identify whether the performer has remediated in a satisfactory way. This evaluation methodology could be utilised within a PASS as one metric to measure the success of the scheme, which, in turn, contributes to the overall evaluation of PASS.

Practical messages:

- It is possible to score a piece of reflective writing using six measures.
- It identifies the metrics to score the writing.
- It can help demonstrate remediation of a performer.

Wider healthcare relevance of the case study:

- Reflection is a skill that everyone should exercise and practice, particularly when learning new skills and embedding learning.
- The logical steps in this evaluation can be applied to any setting where reflection is required.
- Reflection can be used to demonstrate improvement or remediation.

We all need to regularly reflect on our practice in order to be the best that we can. This evaluation methodology could be developed for any piece of reflection and not just for dentists in difficulty. It could be used for self-assessment and developing personal development plans (PDP's).

Table 5.5 Reflective writing evaluation – lessons learned.

Lessons	Changes made (after lesson learned)
It is possible to turn a subjective measure into an objective one that can be measured.	Implementation of a scoring value.
Using the six questions in the methodology wasn't the end of the story when implementing it. It requires development with the mentees to get the most out of it.	A performer who struggles with reflection isn't going to suddenly make the leap to producing an excellent piece without supportive questioning and guidance.
More development and honing to make the methodology simpler to use. There is a difference in reflecting on a CPD course to reflecting when something has gone wrong.	The questions have been altered slightly, as has the way the assessment is introduced to mentees.

Category 3 Case Studies: Early Years in a Dentists' Career

After completion of dental undergraduate education and graduation the vast majority of new dentists in the UK undertake a further year of post graduate training. In Scotland this is known as Dental Vocational Training (DVT), in England, Wales, and Northern Ireland it is known as Dental Foundation Training (DFT). The new dentists spend one year in approved dental practices working with an experienced dentist as their ES in a protected and educational environment developing their skills. They also attend off site tutorials and lectures one day a week to help them reflect on their week whilst consolidating the clinical skills and knowledge they have gained. This year gives the new dentists an introduction into general dentistry and working within the NHS system whilst working in a protected environment. The ES is an important figure who supervises, supports, and guides the new dentist. Throughout the year formative assessment is undertaken and a system of satisfactory completion/review of competence progression is in place. This is a necessary requirement before the new dentist can be placed on the NHS Performers List.

In Scotland completion of the DVT year is necessary before the dentist can be eligible to hold a Health Board (HB) list number which allows the dentist to work in the NHS general dental practice.

'The primary purpose of DFT is to ensure that dentists completing the programme have developed into competent, caring, reflective practitioners who can consistently provide safe and effective care for patients in a primary care setting'. Committee of Postgraduate Dental Deans and Directors (COPDEND) (2015).

Case Study Six: Educational Supervisors and Foundation Dentists

Contributor: Dr. Frederick Fernando BDS

This project is designed to prepare FT's both clinically and psychologically for general practice in the last three months of their foundation year. The protocol aims to ensure a smooth transition and bridge between the foundation year to the working year where the dentist is required to work alone as a general practitioner.

Over the last few years a major trend had been noticed. By early June when foundation dentists realise they have to think about what they would like to do the next year, it seemed as though a 'dark cloud' started to overwhelm them. There is a realisation that for the first time in their career, they will be on their own. There will be no supervisor or clinical demonstrator to look over their shoulder, hold their hand or give them the 'on the spot' advice that they are used to. For some this realisation affects their wellbeing both mentally and physically, causing illness, depression, and anxiety. The issue seemed to be more psychological than clinical. The project was devised to address this very real and worrying issue. By the end of the foundation year, most dentists have had enough experience to enable them to work alone in practice. They will know their strengths and weaknesses but will be able to focus on their weaknesses.

Outline:

- This project is devised to be used by educational supervisors with their designated foundation dentists.
- Designed to prepare the FT both clinically and psychologically for general practice during the last three months of their foundation year.
- The protocol will ensure a smooth transition and bridge between the training year and the working year where one is required to work alone as a general practitioner.
- There is a focus on both coaching and mentoring. The foundation dentist is supported to discover and learn things about themselves in order to achieve and succeed in moving into independent general practice. At the same time, the educational supervisor shares expertise and knowledge, be it clinical but also psychological, in order to support personal and professional growth.

Process:

Stage 1. General Practice Transition Evaluation:
This is a formal meeting, separate to the usual tutorials, between the foundation dentist and their educational supervisor. The meeting will take place in early June, three months before the end of foundation training when the foundation dentist will be applying for jobs. The aim of the meeting is to foster resilience and creativity in the FT by encouraging critical reflection. This is to help increase their self-confidence and reduce any 'fear' they have in moving into general practice. Critical reflection can enable the FT to learn about themselves, others, and their organisations; allowing them to act, based upon a deeper understanding of the complex reality in which they are operating. The critical reflection helps the FT focus on their strengths and gives them the confidence to be ready to work unaided in the next year. During the critical reflection the FT is guided to reflect back on situations they have encountered, forwards to learn from errors and in the present to help them gain confidence. A template is used by the ES to aid the exploration and focus of the conversation. It is important that the FT is encouraged to tell their story, review their situation and determine where they want to get to. Confidentiality is an important ground rule. During the meeting the ES can support the foundation dentist to consider the resources they have at their disposal as they move towards independent practice. These will include physical resources; intellectual resources (for example their clinical skills portfolio), emotional resources, and social resources (for example their friends, colleagues, tutor, and supervisor).

They will also help the FT to explore their values and their future reality. ESs use a scale model to help the FT understand where they are in the present and on a scale of 0–10 how confident and ready they feel they are for general practice. Scale models focus on the positives and what the individual needs to do to achieve a higher number on the scale.

It is expected that this meeting will last approximately two hours. An expected outcome is a plan for how the foundation dentist will prepare during the next three months. The plan is monitored during this time.

Stage 2. Meeting with mentor dentist:
The mentor will be a recently qualified general practitioner about nine months into their career post foundation training. This is the time for the foundation dentist to air any concerns they have about independent practice with the newly qualified general practitioner who has worked for some months in general practice. This is a two-way conversation where the mentor helps to encourage the foundation dentist and dispel any myths which they have about independent practice. It is expected that this meeting will last approximately one hour.

Both meetings aim to help the FT realise their vision, focus on strengths and how to build on strengths.

Evaluation:
Evaluation of the project begins shortly before the FT has completed their foundation year and involves three aspects. One week before completion there is a two-hour meeting between the FT and their ES. The focus of the meeting is on the log and many of the topics raised at the initial meeting will be revisited.

A second meeting takes place one-week post foundation training. This is an hour long informal conversation by telephone between the newly independent dentist and their ES. The focus is to discuss any issues that have arisen and promote learning. Discussion of the plan and goals achieved are an important part. The scale model is repeated to ascertain how confident the dentist is feeling about being independent.

A third meeting takes place three months post foundation training. This is another hour long telephone conversation and repeats the discussions previously had one week after completion of training. After this meeting the process is signed off.

Evaluation of the Educational Supervisor as a Mentor

In addition to evaluation of the process and the foundation dentist it is important to also evaluate the effectiveness of the educational supervisor. This is covered in the exit interview the FT has with their training programme director (TPD). It is at this point that feedback on the ES as a coach and mentor is imperative.

Issues Uncovered During the Process

Issues have come to notice as a result of the project, these can be grouped into three main categories:

- Poor performance
- Communication
- Poor self-awareness.

Poor Performance

There will be situations where both the FT and ES know that the FT may not be fully ready for general practice. Generally, problems can be placed into two major categories, clinical, and non-clinical. If the difficulty is clinical and the FT has self-awareness it is possible to focus on the positives and improve. In these cases, the process circles back to the planning stage. Additional support could include the ES seeing patients of the FT; hands on tutorials; audits.

If the problems are non-clinical and attitudinal then the ES can support the FT to enhance their positive mental attitude and increase belief in themselves. Tools such as Johari window can help the FT to understand their blind spots. Occasionally including the TPD can be helpful.

Communication

Where communication is identified as an issue, it can be worthwhile for the foundation dentist to shadow their educational supervisor, and observe them communicating with patients. Additional study days can provide extra training in communication skills. This could involve scenarios with trained actors, pretending to be difficult patients.

Poor Self-awareness

This is the most difficult situation to deal with. Often the FT believes that they are 'better' than they actually are. Over confidence can be very challenging. During foundation training it is important to encourage confidence but there has to be a self-awareness by the FT that they are inexperienced and have a lot to learn. They may be excellent clinically but may be lacking in interpersonal skills. This may lead to patient complaints.

Some signs to watch out for that could point to a lack of self-awareness include when the FT does not enjoy what they are doing and are only doing it for the accolades and/or money. They may also be taking risks clinically at this early stage of their career.

Practical messages:

- To prepare the FT's both clinically and psychologically for general practice in the last three months of their foundation year.
- The protocol will ensure a smooth transition and bridge the training year into the working year where one is required to work alone as a general practitioner.
- To ensure that the FT's realise they have the ability to work in general practice and to believe in their own abilities.

Wider relevance of the project:

- Believing in ones' own abilities.
- Realising that you have the skills to trust your own judgment.

The system described can be used for general practitioners undergoing PASS or just general dentists who are going through difficult times, whose confidence has been knocked by examples like dental complaints, Legal claims, etc. and so have lost confidence in their own abilities.

Table 5.6 ES and FT – lessons learned.

Lessons	Changes made (after lesson learned)
Knowing that everyone has the ability. We as coaches and mentors need to help the person to trust in themselves.	Implementing the protocol in my day to day FT training with all trainees.
That we as coaches and mentors need to help a person believe in their own judgments.	Following up with the FT regularly to make sure they don't think I have 'abandoned them'. To reiterate what the mentee has learnt from the mentor.

Case Study Seven: Assessing How Coaching and Mentoring Can Impact Dental Students in an Outreach Setting
Contributor: Dr. Stephen Denny BDS

Outreach settings allow dental students to have a taste of dentistry in the real world and outside dental school. Many dental schools now provide sessions of outreach for their students, usually in the fourth and fifth years of training. Most placements are offered in general dental practice, some also take place in community clinics or hospital departments. The dental students attend in small groups and can spend a number of weeks working with a local dental team. Students learn about patient-centred care and providing primary dental care to patients from a variety of social backgrounds. Students develop an appreciation of the responsibilities of the dental team and what it means to work in practice. They develop their clinical skills whilst working with a range of patient groups. Students are supervised closely by senior staff. Students may treat adults and child patients depending on the outreach scheme and they are likely to provide routine examinations, simple restorations, simple endodontics, and extractions.

Southend Outreach Academic Clinic

The dental students who attend the Southend Outreach Academic Clinic are studying at the Institute of Dentistry (IoD) which is one of the six institutes of Barts and the London School of Medicine and Dentistry (SMD), Queen Mary University of London (QMUL).

Outline
Southend outreach opened in 2008. Fourth year dental students attend the outreach one day a week from Whitechapel. Whilst at the clinic students may undertake procedures for the first time. The students must pass 'gateway examinations' during their fourth year to allow them to progress to undertake a wider range of treatments as they progress through their year. All students are assessed on a range of competencies and the treatments they undertake. An electronic system known as 'Liftup' is used to record the marks they achieve. Liftup is generally aligned with the electronic portfolio that foundation dentists complete during their foundation year.

This project aimed to determine the effect that actively developing a coaching and mentoring environment could have on student development and the attitudes to the teaching provided.

The project utilises the Listening Ladder developed by Amy Gaunt (2019, p. 90). In addition, the Spheres of Influence Model (Calluori et al 2003) sets the outline for the project.

Creating the Mentoring Environment – Spheres of Influence

In this model the sphere of influence (Figure 5.2) is composed of four elements:

- **Intention** – of the coach/mentor to be unconditionally supportive to the learning needs, growth, and concerns of the student.
- **Words** – use of words that are non-judgmental and neutral and which allow self-expression of both parties – the coach/mentor and the student.
- **Relationship** – that is free of bias, ego, and 'agenda' on the part of the coach/mentor. The relationship should be inter-developmental.
- **Trust** – this lies at the centre and acts as the glue when the right words, intention, and relationship are present.

The whole sphere of influence increases as any of the circles expand.

Students and tutors were given the diagram and asked which part they felt was the most important. The results were interesting. Here are some of the responses received from students:

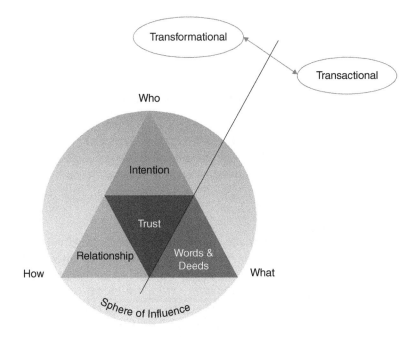

Figure 5.2   Spheres of influence, Calluori & Associates Inc. and The People Factor Inc. (2003).

- 'I feel all of the parts are important – but the "words" part of the diagram is the most important as this is how the other three aspects are communicated to us. How will we know the good intention of the tutor and the level of trust in us without words to help communicate this to us'.
- 'Trust. Trusting the tutors and them trusting you to complete tasks is really good and helps develop confidence'.
- 'I think trust is the most important factor in the diagram'.
- 'When a tutor trusts you, it feels like it is because you are more competent than you believe'.
- 'With trust from the right tutor, I would feel competent in spite of our relationship, their intention, or their words, the other three factors in the diagram'.
- 'I think words underpin everything. I really trust the tutors at Southend because of the way they communicate and give feedback. They challenge me to tackle cases'.
- 'Trust for me is the most important, because if I have trust that the tutor has good intentions and knowledge, I would have more confidence in my practice of dentistry'.
- 'Trust. Because however close the relationship between tutors and students is, whether both parties say the right words or express their intention perfectly lucidly, having trust gives me confidence that we are providing the best possible standard of care to patients. For example, students can trust tutors in making sound clinical decisions, and vice versa tutors trust students to carry out the treatment competently'.

Comments from tutors:

- 'I think words are important as using the correct words should improve relationships and trust. They should also make it clear what the intention is'.
- 'Intention. Us having the intention to improve the students'.
- 'Trust. Once the students trust you generally they are more relaxed and able to tackle more complex procedures'.
- 'Words underpin everything. It nurtures trust, relationships, and shows our intent towards the students'.

An interesting conclusion of the project is that it doesn't really matter which part of the diagram students or tutors felt was the most important because all parts increase the sphere of influence. Engaging in the process and actually discussing things worked. It was positive for everyone to see the results. The students enjoyed having an input and wanted to see the tutors' comments because those comments highlighted that everyone (tutors and students) shared the same goals and objectives.

The students were given a simple questionnaire and an article to read to see how they felt about how they were being taught. We then presented the results to the tutors and students involved. Making simple changes to communication and also to the format of a teaching session has made a huge difference. The aim of the questionnaire was to see how the students scored themselves on their clinical and professional skills (out of 10 1 = low, 10 = high) considering the level of competency they should have achieved when they qualify. Tutors also scored the students and the results of the two groups, students, and tutors was compared. The comparability was good with the students scoring themselves a little higher (range five to seven) and the tutors scoring the students a little lower (range four to seven).

Avoiding words like 'Why?' made a massive impact. The students have valued the feedback more and accepted that feedback is not personal or negative but should promote discussion and help personal development. Examples of comments from students include: 'The feedback and advice from tutors is extremely helpful and encouraging and has really increased my knowledge and improved my clinical abilities. I feel I have learnt more from the tutors here than anywhere else'. 'Excellent feedback. I feel like I have really developed as a clinician while being here – mainly due to the feedback'.

Some students were worried about putting their comments in writing. It was decided to give the students a supervisors' laptop at lunch time to complete the questionnaire. Any identifiers were removed so that the comments were anonymous. Some students were concerned that their responses might be 'wrong'. Most student concerns were reduced after a short introduction into the purpose of the project and the questionnaire.

Observations from patients during the project:
Patient feedback about students was really positive with patients expressing their satisfaction;

- 'Time spent looking after me really good. I was surprised how much care and time the students spent on me'
- 'Treatment first class'
- 'Always explain everything'
- 'Never rushed'

At the end of their placement it was found that all students felt more able to discuss problems with tutors compared with the start of their placement. A very positive finding.

Practical messages:

- Avoid using 'Why did....?'
- Trusting tutors and senior colleagues can have a huge positive impact
- Mentoring is just the way you become, it shouldn't be forced or false. It is positive for everyone involved and helps all sides develop personally and professionally

General observations of the project:

- Feedback is invaluable. Positive feedback breeds confidence and self-esteem.
- Students value tutors trusting them and really value the intentions of the tutors to get them to improve.
- Simple changes to a daily routine make a difference. We now have a student/tutor huddle to chat through things for the day.
- Questionnaire could be rolled out to the whole dental team including DCPs and reception teams and patients.

Table 5.7 Assessing how coaching and mentoring can impact dental students in an outreach setting – lessons learned.

Lessons	Changes made (after lesson learned)
Until you get to know someone and what is going on in their lives I've learnt do not judge or be too harsh.	My daily start has changed. We have huddled in the mornings as open forums. 'What would it look like and feel like to have a great 4th. year?'
Trust is a three-way process. It opens you up to colleagues and students but is hugely rewarding.	Talking more freely. 'What do you need to do or what help do you need to make the next visit even better?'
Trust the process.	The process works. Revisiting course notes has helped.

Wider relevance of the project:

- Why is a negative word, it is much better to replace with 'How could . . ..?', 'How should . . ..?', 'How would. . .?'
- Trust is a fundamental building block to build relationships with students and other team members.
- Once you realise mentoring works and trust the process, then the results follow.

Mentoring should not just be in the dental field. It applies throughout learning and should be in all workplaces.

One year on from the project beginning, the evaluation notes that the general atmosphere has lifted and feels more positive. It feels like a happy learning environment. The outreach clinic has more fun which makes the patients more relaxed and interactive. Communication and support between the tutors, DCP's and reception has improved, however it is recognised that this needs work to maintain.

Case Study Eight: Year 1 Post Foundation Dentists
Contributor: Dr. Keith George BDS

Outline:
The aim of this case study was to put into place an effective mentoring system for year 1 post foundation dentists (Y1PFD) working independently in general dental practice in the NHS. Entering practice from the confines of foundation dentistry offers a major challenge to the still quite recently qualified dentist, it is still a formative period where knowledge, skills, and attitudes acquired are being applied in their practice. It is a major transition period which can be stressful and challenging as well as rewarding. The dentist has no fall back support and could veer off track at this critical time, so this mentoring system was designed to help make the leap. It could be provided in a variety of formats to include face-face, tele-mentoring or via a network. A telephone backup is provided so that the Y1PFD could access help from a mentor. This contact could be anonymous to promote help being sought and reduce any feelings of vulnerability on the part of the early years' dentist.

Table 5.8   Year 1 post foundation dentists – lessons learned.

Lessons	Changes made (after lesson learned)
Lack of scheme at present and minimal support for a scheme.	I have guided this cohort more closely as post graduate dental tutor.
Need for a scheme as litigation against this cohort is large.	
Amount of stress amongst this cohort of dentists.	

Practical messages:

- Give mentees guidance, support.
- Build mentees confidence and act as soundboard for good and bad practice.
- Have someone to answer any questions.

Wider relevance of the project:

- Could be used for any new employees across healthcare although at present most, except dentistry, have it in place.
- Should help patient treatments and experiences.

A scheme to help younger people in whatever field would be beneficial, the mental well-being of them is paramount to everyone and lack of mentoring could lead to mental health issues caused by the stress involved.

Case Study Nine: Smile Restorative Mentoring Programme Contributor: Dr. Jin Vaghela BDS

Outline:

The aim of this mentoring program is to enhance the experience of mentees in their early years as dental associates in General Dental Practice.

Smile Clinic Group (SCG) has prided itself in providing the highest quality dental care to its' patients, through maintaining continuing professional development and supporting its staff to progress in their careers. It strives to create a safe, respectful, and supportive environment that allows both staff and patients to flourish and grow as a family.

SCG employs a number of dentists who have either recently completed DFT or have completed within the last three years.

The dentists at SCG had expressed a need for a programme following DFT to provide continued support with mentoring and study days to reflect on clinical cases and treatment plans. In General dental practice, some of our dental associates may have little opportunity for contact with colleagues when needed and some may work in isolation. It is natural to need support during the early years of practice and primary care dentists can be significantly disadvantaged compared to their hospital counterparts where support is often more easily accessed. The Restorative Mentoring Programme was the response to the need expressed.

Potential obstacles were initially considered to be; time, costs, practicality, and a history of GDP's who had never experienced a mentorship programme.

Studies have also shown a general lack of trained support in General Dental Practice.

Why Mentoring?

It is important to differentiate between mentoring and other educational methods such as teaching, supervision, counselling, therapy, tutoring, and practical placement. A tutor, teacher/educator, or supervisor mainly focuses on promoting and supporting a junior's professional skills, a mentor is an active partner in an ongoing relationship who helps a mentee to maximise his or her potential and to reach personal and professional goals.

The Restorative Mentorship Programme combines a structured one-year modular course along with a two-year mentorship where the early years' dentist has the opportunity to undertake clinical cases in their practice with guidance provided throughout by mentors. During the programme 90 hours of verifiable CPD is provided. Practical worksheets are provided with step by step clinical protocols the dentists can implement in their own practice. In addition, there is a bespoke mentorship day tailored to the individual partnership of mentor and mentee. The day is held at the mentees practice and the mentor and mentee see patients and cases together sharing experience and knowledge.

A maximum number of 17 delegates undertake the programme at any one time.

The following themes and topics are covered during the two years of the programme:

Year 1	Year 2
1) Digital dental photography, digital smile design and tooth whitening.	13) Orthodontics – Quick Straight Teeth (QST).
2) Occlusion in General Dental Practice.	14) Case based discussions and treatment planning.
3) Caries, Anterior and Posterior Composite Restorations.	15) Case based discussions and treatment planning.
4) Anterior Crowns and Veneers.	16) Case based discussions and treatment planning.
5) Posterior Crowns.	17) Case based discussions and treatment planning.
6) Periodontal Treatment – surgical skills.	18) Hands on day.
7) Dentures.	19) Hands on day.
8) Implants and Bridges.	
9) Endodontics.	
10) Tooth surface loss and Onlays.	
11) Complex treatment planning.	
12) Patient management and communication skills.	

A total of 18 case presentations are made during the programme by the early years' dentists.

The Mentors

When recruiting mentors, they are asked to provide a brief biography, together with an outline of the areas in which they would like to mentor, for example; Endodontics, Periodontics, Dental Implants, Prosthodontics, etc. Prospective mentors will also be asked to include information about their approach to mentoring and any preferences they have for meeting arrangements. Due to the geographical distance, this approach works best for the Restorative Mentorship Programme. All mentors are required to have received formal mentor training. Mentoring agreements and ground rules for the relationship are agreed in advance. This will include confidentiality, frequency, timing, and location of meetings, the length of the relationship, goals, aims, and how the relationship will be ended.

Evaluation:

To check that the programme is meeting its aims and fulfilling its true potential, evaluation is an important component.

Online questionnaires are given to all mentors and mentees. In addition, a sample of mentees are selected for individual interviews.

Practical messages:

- Enhance the fitness to practise of dental associates starting in general dental practice.
- Enhance the experience of mentees transitions from DFT to dental associate position.
- Foster a strong community of SCG associates across age groups.

Wider relevance of the project:

Healthcare workers from all professional groups need support, mentors, and to be able to continue to learn and grow.

Dentists operating in all contexts are currently lacking support and access to mentors.

Table 5.9 Smile restoration mentoring programme – lessons learned:.

Lessons	Changes made (after lesson learned)
Structuring a programme for a variety of learning needs.	An ongoing process of evolution.
Costs involved with implementation.	
Monitoring with progression and satisfaction of mentees and our mentors.	

Category Four Case Studies: Risk Management and Quality Assurance (QA)

Risk management is the process by which an organisation identifies, assesses, and controls threats to its' operation. Risks can originate from a variety of sources including individuals. The performance of individuals will have an impact on the success of the organisation.

Individuals who perform well will increase success whilst those who struggle or underperform can decrease success. Systems that can support people to perform well makes good risk management sense. Such systems can operate in two ways, firstly to reduce the factors that can negatively impact on people and secondly to identify and provide support at an early stage to those who are struggling.

QA is the process of ensuring that the correct standards and procedures are in place to produce the desired outcomes. It is part of governance. Methods can include monitoring and inspection, audit, peer review. Mentoring can be an important part of both risk management and QA.

Case Study Ten: Denplan Risk Management/QA (Contributors: Dr. Ewa Rozwadowska BDS and Dr. Catherine Rutland BDS)

Denplan is a dental payment plan specialist, with over 6700 member dentists and around 1.6 million patients across the UK, as well as serving over 2700 companies with employee benefit schemes.

The organisation was set up by two dentists in 1986, with the aim to assist both patients and practice team members with private dental care, offering a range of dental payment plans to suit every oral health need and budget. Denplan is part of Simplyhealth, the UK's biggest cash plan provider.

(Source: www.denplan.co.uk accessed 27.7.20).

In 2016 Denplan invested in Chartered Management Institute (CMI) Level 7 certification in Leadership Coaching and Mentoring training of 12 Advisers. The advisers are dentists with practice appraisal skills who provide practice visits for Excel QA certification. These formally trained coaches and mentors provide a new resource pathway for the risk team to use in order to offer appropriate levels of support to dentists at risk of poor performance.

Within Denplan a number of personnel are involved; to include: consultants (non-dental regional ambassadors); Advisers (dentists who provide certification visits); Advisers and Coach/Mentors; the risk team (co-ordinate risk management); Senior Advisers and the Clinical Director. All these personnel help dentists achieve success by working to develop member dentists' performance – from difficulties to Excel certification. The project describes a coaching and mentoring pathway for the effective use of different groups of individuals to help dentists achieve success

Risks Experienced by Dentists

The organisation has developed a traffic light system to recognise risks and their escalation – red, amber, green (RAG).

The green risk category represents an opportunity for the preventive use of coaching, reducing risk, and growing business safely.

The amber risk category represents possibility. The organisation recognises that supporting practices can help to nudge them back to green.

The red risk category is about supporting practices and dentists. This includes empowering consultants and advisers appropriately, when the risk is identified. Identification

Table 5.10 The Denplan RAG traffic light system.

Green	Amber	Red
Stable practice	Constant change	**Multiple complaints**
Minor concerns – clinical or business related	Clinical and business concerns	**CQC/GDC referrals**
Proactive in intent	Lack of engagement or signs of stress	**Significant health issues**
		Bankruptcy
		Disputes

enables effective referral of cases to the risk team, who can then either deal with the matter themselves, or commission trained coaches and mentors to diagnose the problem correctly and provide the appropriate support.

Denplan has developed and implemented a formalised but flexible coaching and mentoring programme. It is based around Excel certification for standards (see glossary), and provides funding for supporting high risk cases. The programme uses existing expertise at appropriate levels to help dentists run their practices safely.

Practical messages:

- Coaching and mentoring can be used positively to raise standards of all dentists towards the attainment of quality assured certification, whatever their current level of performance.
- The responsiveness of coaching and mentoring services in a large organisation such as Denplan can be leveraged by effectively using the existing resources of Advisers, Consultants, and the senior team.
- Using a positive mentoring approach when supporting dentist members is congruent with 'quality development' both within the profession, as part of the organisational values, and in patient care.

Wider relevance of the case study:

- A coaching and mentoring approach can be used in the development of team members at any level of an organisation. It fosters a collaborative approach to learning, and increases communication channels.
- Coaching and mentoring can support innovative ways of improving patient care through structured QA pathways for clinicians and healthcare teams.
- Coaching and mentoring encourages a positive approach to the development of healthcare teams. This can be incorporated in personal training programmes to help identify and rectify underperformance at an earlier stage.

This case study could be adapted as a framework for using coaching and mentoring in a professional development capacity for both small dental practices and larger organisations for the benefit of patient care.

Table 5.11 The Denplan risk table.

Risk	Consultants	Advisers	Trained Coach/Mentors	Risk Team	Interventions
Red support		Referral to risk team and trained mentors	Formal for risk cases or remediation cases with formalised contracting and agreed outcomes	Information from regulatory bodies or serious internal cases	Remediation Formal intensive C/M of DRiD's/seriously underperforming dentists
Amber possibility	Referral to Advisers via risk team	Information situational coaching/mentoring with industry knowledge and expertise	Formal situational C/M with industry knowledge and expertise	Information from consultants, advisers, and C/M	Formal C/M of cases identified early
Green opportunity	Informal coaching with industry knowledge 'Coaching approach' Training of whole team	Assessment (Excel/FPA)	Light formal C/M for promising new joiners Assessment (Excel/FPA)	Commissioning C/M for new client development	Light formal CM for promising new joiners Assessment (EXCEL/FPA)

Increasing risk and formality

Increasing urgency and seriousness

CM = Coach/Mentoring.
DRiD = Dental registrant in difficulty.

Table 5.12 Denplan risk management – lessons learned.

Lessons	Changes made (after lesson learned)
The role of mentoring to support achievement of the overarching goal of 'quality' to be congruent with patient care assurance, professional performance improvement, and organisational profitability.	Currently implementation phase – no changes measured at present.
The value of training key people in coaching and mentoring to leverage existing resources for raising standards.	
The need for a clear structure for different levels of coaching and mentoring in order to be equitable in the support that can be offered by the company.	

Category Five Case Studies: Tools/Models

There is no shortage of tools and models within mentoring that we can explore and utilise. Megginson and Clutterbuck have published two books that cover techniques and further techniques for coaching and mentoring (2004, 2009). The learning of skills that mentors use in their day to day practice are covered elsewhere in this book. The Forton model is well described in Chapter 4. Tools are what skilled mentors call upon to assist in specific aspects of mentoring and which can be of assistance to particular mentees. Some tools will be of particular help for one person and other tools for another person. A skill of the mentor is in selecting the most appropriate tool for that particular mentee. We hope that the two projects in this section will give you a taste to explore more.

Case Study Eleven: Using Coaching Cards – Tools or Props? Contributor: Ms. Jane Davies-Slowik MBE BDS

Coaching cards can be used to improve communication and develop individuals and teams, supporting the practice of coaching and mentoring. I have used two types of coaching cards, picture cards, and question cards, both of which are available commercially. An alternative is to collect your own favourite postcards and use these with clients instead of commercially available packs. They are easy and fun to use, versatile, and can be a gateway into a previously unexplored area or a deeper coaching conversation.

Picture Cards

Picture cards can be used in a variety of different situations which are described later and are generally used to explore emotions, values, and visioning. They can be used effectively with individuals or teams.

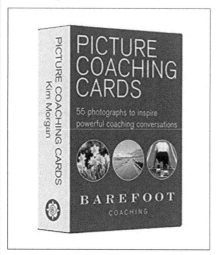

Source: Barefoot Coaching Ltd.

Question Cards

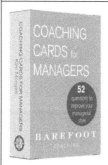 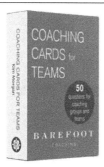 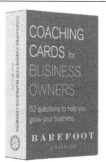 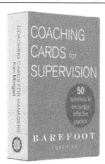

Source: Barefoot Coaching Ltd.

The question cards are written to cover a number of scenarios – for managers, for teams, business owners, and for supervision, as well as for some more day to day coaching exercises

The question cards can be really useful in some situations. Specific packs are available for specific scenarios, for example coaching for managers.

The pack that I like is coaching for supervision and gives some great ideas for starting supervision conversations. They can be really useful for individual reflections for us as coach/mentors.

But they need to be used with caution and should not be a substitute for asking questions out of curiosity after listening to your client.

The Forton Model

- The Principles
  - **Presence**
  - Possibility
  - Partnership
  - **Trust the Client**
  - **Accept, Blend and Create**

- The Skills
  - **Listening**
  - **Reflecting**
  - **Then questioning**

- The Steps
  - **Purpose**
  - **Reality**
  - **Plan**
  - Action
  - **Review**

- The Field
  - Physical
  - Intelectual
  - Emotional
  - Social

Ref: The Forton Group: Professional Leadership Coach Training Programme Student Guide.

Figure 5.3   The Forton group professional leadership coaching model.

The Forton Model of Professional Leadership Coaching (accessed 2020), illustrated in Figure 5.3, describes four domains of coaching. The use of coaching cards can be useful in each of the domains and can be used effectively in team and individual coaching. I find the picture cards most useful so will describe how they can be used in each of the domains.

Domain 1: The Principles of Coaching

One of the mainstays of coaching is the rapport we develop with our clients which helps us to maintain presence for the client. The focus is on the client and their world and the picture coaching cards can help us to understand more about the client's world.

It is vital that we trust the client to be capable and creative and the picture cards allow our clients to use their creativity. Mutual trust is an important skill for leaders as well as mentors, we need to trust our clients to be wise, and to explore insights and perceptions which may emerge from using the coaching cards in a session.

Using the cards will help us to accept blend and create, by using what the client talks about in relation to the picture to explore themes and emotions, blend it with possibility, and create a forward momentum in the client's thinking.

Domain 2: Coaching Skills

Our skills as coaches, listening, reflecting, and questioning, are really important when using the cards. Listening to what the client says, how they describe what they see on the card, how this may be used as a metaphor for something that is happening in their lives, the emotions it provokes, the language they use, their body language, their tone and pace, their thoughts and perceptions are keys to their world.

Reflecting back what we hear our client say can help them to gain deeper insights and we can use coaching questions to deepen the clients' exploration of the situation they are describing in the picture card. The question cards can be used to try out different questions from our usual ones but curiosity about the client and their situation should not be lost.

Domain 3: The Steps

The Forton model (accessed 2020) suggests undertaking the coaching in steps to explore their clients purpose or vision, the reality of their current situation, to plan what action they MIGHT take, developing an action plan, and then review.

The cards can be used during all steps in the coaching conversation, and can be used to explore purpose or their vision, the reality of their current situation, to help to plan options and to review any progress, and to reflect and deepen learning.

Domain 4: The Field, i.e. Resources

The pictures can help to explore the client's resources that they can use to achieve their goals. They can be encouraged to put themselves in the picture or see it from the outside, creating different perspectives which can be used to great effect, particularly if the client feels 'stuck'.

Anthony Gormley – Another Place – Crosby Beach Installation – A Metaphor

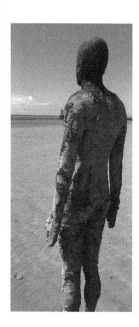

According to Anthony Gormley cited by Richardson (2015, p. 35), his installation of 100 cast iron figures, on Crosby beach, 'Another Place' harnesses the ebb and flow of the tide to explore man's relationship with nature. Each figure modelled on the artists own body has weathered differently.

This is a metaphor for how circumstances, time, and external events, influence our life experience and values in different ways, in much the same way as the elements have transformed these figures.

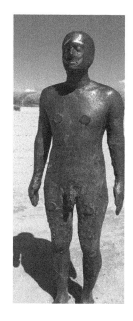

We are all different and have reached the point in our journey as a result of events and life experiences. Coaching is about deepening self-awareness of the resources we already have and need to develop, and the coaching cards can help to do this.

Emotional Intelligence

Coaches help their clients to develop emotional intelligence (EI) and the emotional quotient (EQ) competencies developed by Daniel Goleman (2002), self-awareness, self-management, social awareness, and relationship management can all be explored within a coaching conversation.

Clients' emotions are always present in a coaching interaction and the cards may be a great way of being able to start discussions about emotions. We should be on the lookout for emotional states and attitudes during the session and will be able to explore these particularly when we have excellent rapport with the client.

This might be a way in, to help them to manage their own emotions, recognise emotions in others, and maybe find some strategies to deal with a difficult relationship. A coach can expand their client's awareness of emotion and deepen their capacity to feel what is happening without resisting it.

Coaching for Values

It is really helpful to get in touch with our values to create as little dissonance between our actions and values as possible. When you listen to your client's description of the pictures, you can ask them what is important to them about this? This can help them to get in touch with their values and name them, to explore how particular values are helping them or getting in the way. We should be able to pick up on the values that are important and confirm these with the coachee. This method may also be used in a team coaching situation to align the values of the organisation, the team, and the individual.

Practical Ways of Using Coaching Cards for Team Coaching

Using the picture coaching cards can be handled to great effect in team coaching or team development sessions and could be used with teams in dental practice, groups of trainees, away days, and other team events. The cards can be laid out on a table or the floor and participants invited to choose one which best represents the way they see or feel about the subject which might be in the present, the future, and tell them that they will be invited to say a few words about their feelings or views.

They are great fun to use and people often feel stimulated and able to join in. They can be used as an icebreaker to the session, to assess how people are feeling or what best reflects what they are thinking or at the end of the session as a reflection.

A question could be posed, and team members can pick a card which represents something about their answer to the question and they can talk about it.

Cards can be used for visioning, for example, where do we want to be in five years' time? This will allow discussion of different viewpoints and lead to a shared vision if carefully facilitated by a skilled leader. Goleman (2002) says that under the guidance of an EI leader, people feel a mutual comfort level. They share ideas, learn from one another, make decisions collaboratively and get things done.

Using different cards, comparisons of the future shared vision can be made to the current situation and how different team members see it. This can be used to explore an action plan and what possible changes could be made to take the team or the organisation forward to bring their vision to life.

Values coaching on a team basis may be trickier but some questions about the importance of the subject to individuals can open up discussions on shared values and lead to more resonance within the team.

The cards can be useful as a wrap up exercise – how did the session go? what new insights do team members have?

Practical Ways of Using Coaching Cards for Individual Coaching

Coaching cards can be used very powerfully during a one to one coaching session. They can be used to great effect for exploring visioning and reality and values coaching. It helps us as coaches to get into the client's world and we can gather useful information about the client, their emotional state and their communication preferences. Let your coachee choose a card or cards and encourage them talk about them or ask them a coaching question to stimulate their thought processes.

The use of cards depersonalises the situation and may help the client talk about difficult emotions and also encourages creativity and imagination which can really help to make the sessions fun, interactive, and illuminating.

The cards can also be used to give feedback for example from the coachee to us as coaches.

Shirley Gaston (2014) summarises a variety of ways of using picture cards in group or individual sessions for the following reasons:

- Tap into personal experiences and feelings.
- Understand a variety of perspectives.
- Have private time to reflect before sharing with the group.
- Seek patterns and make connections.
- Elicit stories and create metaphors.
- Articulate what is known to the group.
- Articulate what has been unspoken or 'undiscussable'.
- Create dialog.
- Build on ideas.
- Explore complex issues.
- Imagine alternatives.
- Spark humour and playfulness.
- Transfer learning into new situations.

She suggests questions that can be posed in different circumstances such as asking an individual to choose a card that represents what they want to achieve at the end of a session or as a life goal, a useful resource. The cards can be used to explore how people are feeling about their current situation or about future options and in team coaching may be the route to understanding different perspectives from different members of the team and to develop shared values or a shared vision.

Self-development

Both picture and question cards can be used as a vehicle for self-development, to explore our thoughts and deepen self-awareness.

Conclusion

Both picture and coaching cards can be used during coaching sessions with individuals and teams and can also aid self-reflection for us as coaches. They can be used in many different ways at different stages of the coaching conversation.

They are not a substitute for excellent coaching skills and should be used as tools not props to support our coaching rather than as a substitute for curiosity, and great listening and questioning skills.

Practical messages:

1) Coaching cards are really useful tools but should never be used as a substitute for intelligent and intuitive coaching.
2) Coaching cards can be used in a number of different scenarios with individuals and teams, to explore sometimes complex issues and deepen the individual or team's self-awareness.
3) Sets of coaching cards can be bought or you can have fun collecting your own to use.

Table 5.13 Using coaching cards – lessons learned.

Lessons	Changes made (after lesson learned)
People enjoy the exercise and are usually keen to voice their thoughts and tend not to be intimidated by the exercise.	Give everyone time and space to say as much or as little as they are willing to.
Sometimes unexpected thoughts and feelings emerge from the exercise.	Leave time for the individual to articulate what they want to say and how they are feeling. Use of silence is important to allow for individuals speed of thought processing. Use questions to deepen the awareness. Go with the client and explore their feelings and metaphors with them.
Picture cards are enjoyable but sometimes question cards offer a different stimulation.	On occasions use question cards particularly if the individual feels stuck.
The picture cards can be used to explore issues from different perspectives.	Ask the coachee to step inside the picture and explore how that is for them, then ask the coachee to look at the picture from a different perspective, e.g. a member of their family, their boss, etc.

Wider Relevance:

1) Picture coaching cards can be used during practice or team development days as a fun and interesting way of exploring ideas from different perspectives or during individual conversations with staff.
2) Question cards could be used for team meetings but to be used sparingly.
3) For individual staff development and in leading the dental team.

Case Study Twelve
Contributor: Mrs. Shilpa Chitnis BDS

Outline

My **P.E.A.R.L.S.** of communication is a strategic step-by-step model which helps the user to understand the importance of effective communication to enhance an individual's performance. The steps can be replicated in different facets of the dental environment and are practical and easy to apply with self-explanatory steps.

- **P – PERSPECTIVE**
- **E – EMPATHY**
- **A – AWARENESS**
- **R – RAPPORT**
- **L – LISTENING**
- **S – SUPPORT**

P – PERSPECTIVE

Perspective is an outlook or interpretation about any given situation or topic. It is *a point of view* which is usually affected by our conditioning, life experiences, and expectations. We view things the way our thoughts want us to and this is affected by our focus at that point in time. However, it is worth remembering that if we change the way we look at things, the things we look at change too.

For example: I'm running late and treating an extremely irritable patient and feeling agitated and awkward. This is provoked by the dental nurse being extremely slow preparing the instruments for the crown preparation appointment. My mood prompted me to be abrupt and abrasive with the dental nurse, as I felt she was being unfocused. My actions led her to become defensive, which created an uncomfortable atmosphere between us, whilst continuing to remain professional in front of the patient. We both had our own opinions of the situation during the *stand-off* and this led to us both being judgemental towards each other. This in turn resulted in different conflict reactions, from an emotional outburst versus withdrawing and no communication.

When we are open and take notice of different perspectives, we will naturally be more accommodating and improve our communication skills.

E – EMPATHY

Empathy lies in our ability to understand and share the feelings or situation of another and is a skill which can be learnt and improved upon. It is an important factor contributing to

EI (also known as emotional quotient or EQ) which is the ability to understand, use, and manage our own emotions in positive ways to relieve stress, communicate effectively, empathise with others, overcome challenges, and defuse conflict. Empathy creates a bond and improves communication by building trust. We are more likely to trust someone that we believe understands us and our point of view. Expressing or showing empathy is intuitive for some, while with others it takes conscious effort. In my experience, we are either predominantly *task-oriented* or *people-oriented*, whilst a few can fall into both categories.

Considering these attributes brings to mind two dentists, Alice and Carole, who work in partnership with each other and were keen to maximise their communication skills. Alice felt that Carole could be insensitive and blunt in her communication style. Carole, although very conscientious, could express herself as being aloof and reserved. Carole found it difficult to initiate conversation and so it was difficult for her to talk about anything other than the treatment plan with her patients. She also struggled to say 'no', which resulted in appointment disarray and left her frustrated after *assuming* she was being criticised by both staff and patients for the practices' timetabling. With the support of a mentor Carole was able to take the first step towards learning the skill of empathy. By firstly being kinder to herself, it created a ripple effect to people that she came into contact with.

Kindness of ourselves gives us the ability to understand the other person's situation and/or feelings, which subsequently enables them to trust the person who is being empathetic.

Empathy is a building block for any relationship to improve and flourish upon.

A – AWARENESS

Self-awareness is the ability to focus on ourselves and how our actions, thoughts, or emotions do or do not align with our internal standards.

To self-improve can be difficult to achieve as we need to remain objective and present. We are creatures of habit and often work on *autopilot* which does not necessarily lend itself well to helping us to reach our full potential.

Awareness of others. This skill is the ability to be empathetic. We *tune* in to the emotions or feelings of others which helps us with insight into their strengths and weaknesses and reflects on the way we communicate. Irrespective of verbal or non-verbal communication, the recipient will feel the connection, which in turn helps build trust.

Impact of Self on Others and Impact of Others on Self. This form of awareness helps us in the way we conduct ourselves. By this I mean the way we *respond* rather than *react*. Being aware of the impact on the situation enables us to be *resilient* rather than *temperamental*. This results in a viable and open communication which leads to a positive end result.

R – RAPPORT

Being *interested* rather than being *interesting* is the first step in building rapport. Being genuinely interested in the other person helps create an honest connection. Building rapport is like building a connection which includes trust, confidence, and ease of communication.

When we begin with open-mindedness and a kind heart, establishing rapport naturally follows. When we find rapport with someone, there is clarity in our communication with them.

Consider task-oriented individuals. They should not be interpreted as being insensitive just because they are driven by *doing*, which can take precedence over them being emotive. However, individuals who are people-oriented, are clearly more *naturally* aligned towards rapport. For those individuals where rapport is more natural, it is difficult for them to understand why it isn't for others.

When I was in the process of creating the P.E.A.R.L.S model, it was very apparent to me that rapport is the main ingredient to achieve a positive result with both team communication and patient treatment acceptance. If my mentee and I share an excellent rapport, they will be more likely to share their vulnerability and access their blind spot, which results in us both maximising our growth potential. If the mentee openly shares their fears, this will lead to them being able to explore opportunities which will likely be out of their comfort zone. Having an open and non-judgmental environment is an important aspect which helps bring this to fruition.

In my experience it is easier for me to trust my mentor who is *authentic* and *approachable*, and this is only achieved by the way in which we communicate and conduct ourselves.

L – LISTENING

Good communication starts with active listening. And by listening, I mean to understand rather than to reply. When we actively listen, we listen for words as well as feelings. Often when we listen, we are influenced by our own biases and so we listen to answer and to put in our views and so actually miss what is being said.

Active listening is a skill which can be refined. It is important to do so, as it helps build trust and respect and supports rapport and connection. Active listening also helps avoid miscommunication and misunderstanding which avoids and/or resolves conflict. Active listening is *the* key element in effective communication.

For a successful coaching/mentoring relationship it is important to ask open-ended questions and even more important, active listening gives the mentee time to process and then speak. We all process information differently and our own conditioning affects the interpretation. As a part of the mentoring process, I have learnt the power of pause/silence. Silence can be awkward for most people and our reaction is to fill the silence. But we must be mindful that silence holds crucial information, opportunities, and possibilities for the mentor and mentee.

Using *encouragers* like the word 'and' is powerful, as it can stimulate the mentee to expand and think *outside of the box*. The process of open questioning, with patient, active listening inspires the mentee to reach their blind spots and their unexplored strengths and opportunities. This strategy often results in the mentee disclosing useful information without being aware.

As much as listening to the spoken word, a good mentor or coach is the one who can help the mentee feel comfortable enough to open up and divulge things which they ordinarily would not be able to put into words. It helps the mentor be confident to achieve the goal they are setting, or alternatively find a solution to the problem or concern they are facing.

Using the pause/silence approach, while the mentee is processing their sentences or thoughts, is important, to be highly valued and **not** to be interrupted. When we are fearful, we are reluctant to share our mind unless it is with a person we trust and respect. As an empathetic and rapport building mentor, to be able to develop trust and respect is key in enabling the mentee to share their inhibitions and vulnerabilities and to overcome this by reaching their true potential.

When we are completely present, the listening will be an easier process.

S – SUPPORT

Support is about getting help and advice consistently to keep achieving your goals, whilst working with focus on all aspects of growth (i.e. personal or professional) support can be from a team of people close to us, family and friends, or co-workers, coaches and/or mentors.

Support of a great team is paramount in dividing the task to multiply the success. The strength of the team is in the strength of the individual members. By supporting every individual within your team by building each other up, it will inspire and build a passionate team all working towards the same vision.

The people we have around us will influence our thoughts and actions and so it is important to have the support of people who can bring out the best in us and keep us in a positive frame of mind. This encourages and stimulates a growth mind set.

It is often a struggle for us to ask for help and this is due to our own inhibitions and fears. Fear of being judged and fear of failure are the obstacles which stop us from taking steps towards achieving our goals. This leads to procrastination and we become stressed and overwhelmed. By asking for help we get to see our unseen opportunities (or access to our blind spots.) It also boosts our mental well-being.

In summary, the P.E.A.R.L.S model (Figure 5.4) is relevant in all aspects of life where communication is prevalent. To become well versed in this strategy, naturally results in more P.E.A.R.L.S. (treasures) being activated in our lives.

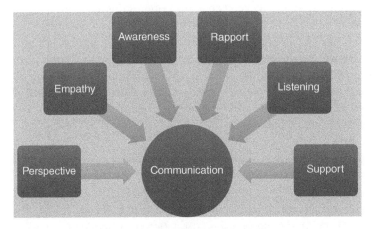

Figure 5.4 P.E.A.R.L.S. – a model for communication.

Practical messages:

- Remain open in challenging circumstances. ***Consider the other point of view***
- Value different opinions and review constructively. ***Trigger your growth mind set.***
- Be kind in actions and words. ***Create positivity around you.***
- Understand rather than assume. Avoid your assumption leading to miscommunication.
- We process things, thoughts, and feelings differently. ***Respect each other's differences.***
- Always ask for help when we cannot see a way forward. ***This is a strength, not a weakness.***

Lessons learnt:

- ***Understanding*** the different aspects of communication enables us to focus on our outward conduct to others.
- ***Respond*** rather than ***react*** remains a constant 'work in progress'.
- ***Respect*** in conflict results in resolution and closure.
- ***Actively*** listening triggers more patience.
- ***Kindness*** to you and me is essential for self-preservation and resilience.
- ***Focus*** our efforts on being non-judgmental.
- Take time to ***reflect.***
- ***Summarise*** all communication to achieve clarity, which improves listening skills and decreases miscommunication.
- ***Support*** is the biggest reward. Both in helping others and asking for help.

Communication is simply the act of transferring information from one person or group to another.

Every communication involves (at least) one sender, a message, and a recipient. This may sound simple, but communication is clearly a complex subject. The transmission of the message from sender to recipient can be affected by a huge range of things, these include our emotions, the cultural situation, the medium used to communicate and even our location.

P.E.A.R.L.S creates a positive environment in which good communication can thrive.

The complexity of communication is why good communication skills are considered so desirable by employers around the world: accurate, effective, and unambiguous communication is actually extremely hard. I therefore hope that you have enjoyed my P.E.A.R.L.S. of wisdom as much as I did in writing them.

We would like to acknowledge the kind participation and contributions of all our colleagues who generously shared the projects they have developed. Their case studies have been included to help the profession to benefit from their experiences of introducing and using coaching and mentoring within dentistry.

References

Calluori & Associates Inc. and The People Factor Inc. (2003). Spheres of Influence.

Committee of Postgraduate Dental Deans and Directors (2015). *Dental Foundation Training Curriculum*. UK: COPDEND.

Committee on Standards in Public Life (1995). The seven principles of public life (the Nolan Principles). www.gov.uk accessed 29 April 2020).

Department of Health (2000). *Modernising NHS Dentistry – Implementing the NHS Plan*. London: Department of Health.

Forton Group Limited, (2002). The professional leadership coaching model. https://thefortongroup.com/93-about-us/faq/284-what-is-the-professional-leadership-coach-model Accessed 4 June 20

Gaston, S., (2014). 10 ways to use picture cards in your workshops and coaching sessions https://www.linkedin.com/pulse/20140612101813-1905000-10-ways-to-use-picture-cards-in-your-workshops-and-coaching-sessions/ accessed 5 June 20

Gaunt, A. and Stott, A. (2019). *Transform Teaching and Learning Through Talk. The Oracy Imperative*. Rowman and Littlefield.

General Dental Council (2017). *Shifting the Balance: A Better, Fairer System of Dental Regulation*. GDC.

Goleman, D., Boyatziz, R., and McKee, A. (2002). *The New Leaders. Transforming the Art of Leadership into the Science of Results*. Sphere publishers.

Megginson, D., Clutterbuck, D. (2004). Techniques for Coaching and Mentoring. Blackwells

Megginson, D., Clutterbuck, D. (2009). Further Techniques for Coaching and Mentoring. Blackwells

National Guardian's Office (2019). Freedom to Speak up. Guidance for NHS Trust and NHS Foundation Trust Boards. Publications code: CG44/19.

Regulation of Dental Services Programme Board (2015). The future of dental service regulation. cqc.org.uk

Regulation of Dental Services Programme Board (2017). Operational Protocol. Working together to reduce duplication. A practical guide for staff. V2.0. NHS England Publications Gateway ref. 07432.

Richardson, T. (2015). *Walking Inside Out: Contemporary British Psychogeography*. Rowman & Littlefield International.

Taylor, M., Purdue, D., Wilson, M., and Wilde, P., (2005). Evaluating community projects. Joseph Rowntree Foundation, York.

UK Caldicot Guardian Council (2017). A Manual for Caldicott Guardians. https://www.gov.uk/government/groups/uk-caldicott-guardian-council

6

Discussion

This chapter brings together some of the emerging themes from the case studies and explores them in more depth. Topics that have their roots in professional mentoring are also included. The discussion is not meant to provide definitive answers but to expand the issues and promote reflection. The aim is to provoke thinking.

The book was written with the intention of showcasing practical applications of mentoring within dentistry in the UK. We feel it's time to stop paying lip service to mentoring, coaching, and reflective practise. The time is right to re-energise these core skills and ensure they form a solid foundation for quality relationships within the profession. In this way, the authors believe standards will be raised at individual, practice, and organisational levels, across the profession. We believe that many of the lessons learned here are also applicable across the wider healthcare professions as well.

To quote the EMCC (2020): 'Coaching is the best methodology to create awareness about any resistance for change. ... Mentoring has proven to be an effective catalyst for change...'

The dental profession has so much to offer; yet sometimes it can appear that its' status and power is diminished as the 'Cinderella' service in health prevention, treatment, and care. The global pandemic of Covid-19 has illuminated the considerable strengths, flexibility, and transferable skills of dentistry, as well as the significant demands placed upon it.

Talking with medical professionals on the front line of emergency care shows how important it is for everyone to stay focused in their use of PPE: hour after hour. Dental professionals redeployed during the first wave of the pandemic have proved themselves to be exemplary in this area because it's an approach to practise that they are well used to. Their focus and attention to detail make them role models for systematic application of PPE, with a detailed focus on its correct use in different situations.

This is an argument for coaches and mentors to spread their wings outside the profession, as well as raising standards within it. The factors described in the case studies, for example, are not solely confined to the domain of dentistry. We argue that dental professionals benefit greatly from shared learning across the wider health sectors, and wider coaching and mentoring professions and vice versa. This is reflected in our own experience of delivering education and training. The case studies also show how much the profession has

Practical Applications of Coaching and Mentoring in Dentistry, First Edition.
Janine Brooks and Helen Caton-Hughes.
© 2021 John Wiley & Sons Ltd. Published 2021 by John Wiley & Sons Ltd.

to offer the wider coaching and mentoring community; for example, the topic of the six measurable steps of reflective practice in case study five.

By achieving recognised qualifications or credentials, such as the Post Graduate Certificate (from awarding bodies such as the CMI or the ILM) or from the ICF, dental professionals can apply their skills in other fields too. The more academic options (e.g. CMI, ILM) support the critical thinking relevant to the development of a mentoring and coaching service to professional standards; helping define policy and support the professionalism which the GDC demands. ICF and similar credentials focus more on the skills of a coach and their practical application. For dental professionals looking at coaching and mentoring as a future career option, or as part of their professional portfolio, these routes are flexible and not mutually-exclusive, which supports better career choices.

Beyond One-to-One: Coaching and Mentoring Groups and Teams

Over the years delivering training in coaching and mentoring, we invite participants to plan how they will apply these skills, and to reflect on how they best work in the professional environment.

While coaching or mentoring may have started as a dialogue between two people, it quickly became much more: whether reflecting the greater need for communication, collaboration, and alignment between colleagues. Taking into account financial drivers, one to many coaching and mentoring sessions are now an accepted format.

Group Coaching and Mentoring

Group coaching and mentoring is for people who aren't necessarily part of the same organisation or team, although they can be. They do not share, necessarily, the same personal goals, but come together to benefit from the coaching and mentoring experience.

For example, a group of dental professionals may have the profession in common yet have very different career aspirations: to take their careers forward in speciality, practice ownership or corporate environments. In these situations, group coaching can be a way of validating, acknowledging, and supporting peoples' aspirations – especially if there is no family or cultural background in the profession. Coaching questions can support people to focus on their goals, values, and development gaps, to help them make those aspirations a reality.

Group mentoring can offer real-life examples and ideas for ways to grow an individual's career; for people to share ideas and explore the pros and cons.

Group sessions also support peer learning: providing the peer motivation and encouragement that a one-to-one session lacks.

Group coaching and mentoring is a valuable experience particularly as a way to introduce people to the concepts and experience of coaching/mentoring. Taster sessions in groups like this help demonstrate that it's possible to discuss even sensitive subjects in a safe space. Focused on individual aspirations and goals more than team coaching (discussed below), in our experience, many people who first encounter coaching or mentoring in a group, find it easier to ask for one-to-one support too, and to work better in teams where coaching and mentoring is offered.

Team Coaching and Mentoring: Shared Goals and Direction

Team coaching refers to people who share a common task, goal or direction; whether they work together in the same location, share a common boss, or are coming together for a project, with the intention of achieving a specific goal.

Less focused on individual aspirations than group coaching or mentoring, team coaching also involves leadership: its vision, shared values, and team development. The power of the team can be unleashed when coaching, using reflective practise and action learning, and all can turn aspirations into a successful reality.

Often, while teams talk the rhetoric of 'plan, do, review' for team projects, most of the time is spent 'doing' with the plan phase under-valued and the 'review' stage reserved for exploring 'what went wrong and who's to blame?'

Team coaching and mentoring is an investment in future success; it helps pull the team together and head towards the goal, as well as creating a strong bond between team members.

Team coaching is, however, a specialist coaching and mentoring activity, demanding an understanding of team dynamics, and balancing the tasks with the team's social cohesion and an understanding of leadership coaching – such that every member of the team realises their potential.

For example, collaboration and communications are easy terms to pay lip service to, yet team coaching needs to address issues like co-operation versus competition; the giving or withholding of information; shared plans, lived values, and so on.

Team mentoring gives team members the opportunity to get help and support for their roles, but sometimes it takes courage to do this in a team environment. Where bosses or managers lead by example, and are transparent about their own involvement with coaching and mentoring, team members find it easier to engage with these activities.

Coaching in Virtual Environments

The sudden transfer to virtual environments, such as 'voice over internet' audio or video calls, during the initial stages of the COVID-19 pandemic, hastened the already-popular use of these systems for coaching and mentoring.

In the days before video calling was ubiquitous, many coaches would say that they had never 'met' their coaching clients in person. Face to face meetings, whilst desirable, are not essential in the mentoring/coaching process. The skills of receptive listening, reflecting, asking questions, and offering support do not demand in-person meetings, and coaching is highly effective without them.

Mentoring benefits from in-person contact, with activities like work-shadowing, demonstrating technique or other activities – although Soumya and Ramachandra (2011) tell us that 'technological advances are helping change the way students learn'. The haptics technology allows students not only to 'treat a virtual patient', but also to receive objective feedback about the procedure during and after the 'treatment session'. 'Virtual environments are impacting traditional methods of direct contact mentoring and methods of delivery'. This also depends on the particular type of mentoring that is provided. For example, in our experience career mentoring can be successfully provided using remote methods.

What people value most is the empathy, trust, and safety of the coaching and mentoring conversations; the feeling that someone believes in their capabilities and potential. These are not confined to in-person conversations, and can be built in other ways – both visually and by telephone.

Coaching in Organisations: Organisational Dynamics, Does Size Matter?

The dental profession has changed dramatically in recent years. It reflects four global revolutions in technological advancement: in information technology (IT), energy, manufacturing, and the wider Life Sciences sector. Not forgetting the rise in dental bodies corporate. Each of these revolutions will impact the dental profession in some way, and probably more rapidly than we think. For example, new methods of manufacturing, such as 3D printing, has already arrived in many dental technician laboratories and dental practices, which in turn creates a focus on the costs of, and access to, energy.

Since the expansion of the dental corporates in the UK, the definition of what it means to be a dental practice has also changed radically. Whilst the possibility of improved purchasing power and capital investment makes these organisations more viable, the risk is the loss of personalised care and the influence on professional autonomy.

Coaching to develop people skills and improve staff management; to create better leaders are all possible within the organisational coaching context. Supporting people to see that today's leadership now comes from influence, rather than control; that there is more than one agenda at play – with competing priorities – makes leadership and management more confusing. Many dental professionals, used to the traditional practice working environment, may struggle with this shift in focus and priorities; coaching and mentoring to support people through change is a key intervention.

Coaching and Mentoring Boundaries

Coaching and mentoring has the potential to raise standards at individual, practice, and organisational levels, yet there are boundaries to consider and these interventions are not a magic solution to every issue.

For example, coaching a member of staff is not a substitute for a manager's clear target setting, performance management, and direction. Nor does it absolve anyone of communicating clear information or taking difficult decisions. A coach or mentor may support the thinking process behind a decision, but the responsibility for taking, and communicating, a decision, lies with the coachee/mentee themselves.

Some writers, e.g. Goleman et al. (2002) describe coaching as a 'leadership style' and the authors themselves teach coaching for managers to use it as an additional skill set to improve people-management behaviours.

But there are times when coaching or mentoring are not appropriate: for example, the ICF identifies the imbalance of power between a manager and a direct report. In this situation, where there are common drivers, whether that's a financial target, a deadline or a rulebook; there may be conflicts of interest. This means that managers can be 'coach-like' but are not operating as independent, objective, professional coaches.

The good news is that dental professionals are typically used to reflecting on ethical issues and potential, or actual, conflicts of interest. Knowing one's own professional boundaries – what one is trained, equipped, qualified, and experienced to do – makes it easier to identify those activities outside of one's competence.

The typical discussion area we cover in our training programmes are the boundaries between the therapeutic talking professions, such as counselling, psychotherapy, and so on, and coaching and mentoring. The simple response is that coaching is rooted in the recent past and the present, with an emphasis on desired future outcomes. It does not typically explore the distant past (e.g. 'childhood'), but may use the past to find examples of issues and challenges to change future behaviours. Mentoring uses the past as a valuable resource of personal and professional experience on the part of the mentor with the hope that this may be of value to the mentee in the future.

Good mental health and wellbeing is vital, and many coaching and mentoring clients will also seek support from mental health professionals, at the same time as pursuing a coaching programme. The two are not mutually-exclusive.

What our coaching and mentoring students often express is a concern that 'coaching for emotions' is akin to therapy. There's a key distinction to be made here: when we are receptively listening to people, that's a natural human behaviour. The training we receive to listen well and be open and receptive to others is an enhancement of something we already do, quite regularly, and naturally. Whenever we discuss things of importance, we'll share details. We'll also share how we feel about the topic. We may also speculate on how others are feeling too. Again, these are all natural parts of a normal, everyday conversation.

Learning coaching and mentoring skills is simply using our receptivity, our listening skills, our presence, our supportive attitude, to pay extra attention to what someone is trying to achieve, through what they are saying (and how they say it). It may feel like a great conversation, boosting confidence; we may feel like we are expressing anger, frustration or other concerns – because our emotions are engaged in the conversation. Learning to be a better coach or mentor is simply learning how to engage, positively, with other peoples' feelings and help them see how these are having an impact – whether for good or otherwise. It's a powerful and extremely helpful skill to develop, without crossing any professional boundaries.

This is not to say that, when creating a coaching and mentoring policy, we do not address the risk management issues; see case study ten, for an example of the thinking on this topic. Case studies one and nine also address the issue of the boundaries of coaching and mentoring, in their situations and context.

How and When to Use Coaching and Mentoring

Whether delivered in groups, teams or one-to-one, coaching, and mentoring enables professional growth through personalised learning. This means that it can be used at different times during a career, and in different ways, as the case studies show.

Over the last 20 years, the authors have identified a range of different situations where coaching and mentoring have been used successfully, some elements that support these conversations and some of the barriers that prevent them.

Word of mouth has been the single most powerful driver of coaching and mentoring: when someone experiences for themselves the benefits of having someone to take their goals, aspirations – and fears – seriously, and helps them find solutions, it can be a life-changing experience. However, there are signs of a slow uptake of coaching and mentoring in the dental profession; see case study four, for example. The question arises of whether training in this field seems less relevant or tangible to dental professionals, who prefer CPD in technical or clinical fields and find it easier to see the relevance of those CPD activities. Or whether this is because dental professionals find it hard to ask for help, and perhaps doing that is stigmatised within the profession. Another possibility could be that we need to sharpen up our application and understanding of the term 'mentoring'. Traditional understanding of mentoring as being the passing of knowledge and skill from one experienced practitioner to another could be interpreted as mentoring being simply giving advice. If this is the interpretation, then almost any experienced practitioner can be a mentor. Modern mentoring is so much more than giving advice, in fact that aspect has taken a back seat to the other skills that trained mentors can bring to a relationship. We need to value mentors and mentoring and not assume the role can be automatically undertaken without additional skills training.

It is as important to understand when and where coaching and/or mentoring might be relevant and helpful, as it is to know how to provide coaching and mentoring services well. The calls from within the profession for structured 'peer support', that offers skilled guidance at the local level, help set the framework for its greater use.

The role of professional organisations, like the ICF, Association of Coaching and EMCC, or qualification bodies, like the CMI or ILM in the UK, or universities that both teach coaching and mentoring *and* make it available to their own staff, have all helped define and shape the coaching and mentoring professions, making it accessible to a wider range of people and identifying what makes it work so well.

The rise of neuroscience has played its part too, as people understand the brain better, and appreciate how it learns. While our reptilian brain operates out of fear, or to fulfil immediate desires, our mammalian brain helps us nurture ourselves and others. It's in this part of our brain – the 'meaning making machine' combining our rational thinking and our feelings – that deeper learning becomes embedded.

By creating learning cultures in organisations that celebrate reflective practice, productive conversations, and collaborative communication, we can all create a higher performance and learning environment for everyone.

Barriers to Introducing Coaching and Mentoring

Attitudinal Barriers

At their very best, dental teams are made up of highly qualified and well-trained clinicians, support staff with people and practical skills and well-run administrative systems. Yet these very systems and skills can be a barrier to personal and professional development.

If someone believes they 'should' be able to cope – despite the major and volatile change in today's world, they will create their own barrier to seeking help and support. One theme arising across the case studies, is that of prevention, as well as early detection and addressing of issues of concern. Case studies six and seven particularly, consider these issues of prevention and supportive development.

If a fellow professional believes themselves and their colleagues 'shouldn't fail', the support that is available will not be widely shared as a resource – whether through internal communication systems, or by word of mouth.

The introduction of coaching and mentoring services is not just about the practical organisational tasks, it's also about the attitudes to these types of services. As a profession, dentistry needs to get past these outdated attitudes. To remove current stigmas around seeking help, a change of attitude is needed.

There's also a positive element to this issue. Coaching and mentoring is not just about prevention of poor service, remediation when things go wrong or development to improve practise; it's also about excellence.

Taking a positive approach is also the best way to break down stereotypes: whether that's attitudes towards one part of the dental team, towards women, or people of colour. Holding limiting beliefs about peoples' potential will hold back the whole team. Supporting up-skilling across the team through career development plans for all our colleagues will naturally address traditional stereotyping. We're none of us immune to bias, but we can look beyond the labels we place on ourselves and colleagues and move forward faster and more effectively.

At a time of rapid change in technology and life-sciences, we can all play a part in developing new ways to improve peoples' health and prevent disease; make treatments easier and more appealing and reduce the challenges and burdens of working within the dental profession that currently arise.

As a result of this innovation, new opportunities will arise for dental professionals to expand their skill base and work in new ways.

Structural Barriers

Having policies and systems that support coaching and mentoring is the first, most important step to removing structural barriers to coaching. Another typical barrier is finance: the fear of the cost of such programmes. While the evidence exists to demonstrate extremely high value returns on investment in coaching and mentoring, this barrier still remains.

Typical Benefits of Coaching and Mentoring

In our own unpublished findings (Forton 2020), for clients that have introduced a 'coaching culture', that is, have trained a number of people in coaching and mentoring skills to a suitable standard inside the organisation (with or without their achieving credentials or qualifications), a range of typical benefits have been identified:

- Recruitment and retention benefits – for example by providing induction programmes that include coaching and mentoring.

- Leadership development benefits – in the healthcare sector, the number of managers from medical backgrounds passed their leadership training sooner with coaching support.
- Cost savings – identifying – and winning – new income streams, cutting internal, and external costs, reducing overheads.
- Reductions in 'grievances' and employment litigation.
- Improved health and safety (e.g. measured by number of incident-free days).
- Faster achievement of team and project goals, without loss of quality or 'cutting corners'.

The case studies support reflective practise, self-awareness, and critical thinking – all vital for independent professionals. The goals include helping reduce complaints and litigation, especially those career-defining incidents that can easily be prevented, thus saving time, emotional strain, and money.

Impact of Coaching and Mentoring

Prevention

A consistent theme across the case studies is the impact of prevention of a range of issues, by, for example, raising awareness of the need for high standards, and by the early detection of – and addressing – issues quickly.

Neutralising

Coaching and mentoring can be used to reduce internal and external threats. Internally, it can de-escalate conflict, which reduces management and human resource time, and the potential for legal costs. An external example is patient complaints, which not only cost time and money but drain people's morale. Preventing and neutralising complaints improves staff and patient relationships.

Remediation

Everyone makes mistakes and coaching and mentoring can support fitness to practise issues and remediation, when the individual recognises, and is willing to act and make change. Mentoring can support the 'how to' and coaching approaches support reflective practice, or the 'why'.

Performance Conversation

One of the conversations that supervisors, leaders, and managers find hardest, is to give constructive support and feedback. Learning to listen to staff members, encouraging reflection, and supporting success can have dramatic improvements and both coaching and mentoring approaches support this.

Development Conversation

Part of every performance conversation should include development, with the aim of achieving excellence. This is not just for the benefit of the individual, although taking an interest in people's career goals supports engagement and loyalty, it has a business benefit too. Supporting people to see career options, whether to specialise or generalise, whether to stay in a clinical field or branch off into non-clinical roles, these will all play to an individual's strengths and are more likely to inspire motivation, innovation, and commitment.

Themes from the Case Studies

The following section reviews and shines a light on some of the key themes to emerge from the case studies. Whilst each case study describes a unique project they share some important messages. We have highlighted some take away messages from each theme at the end of each section.

Personal Performance

Several case studies described centre around PASS. As already noted there has been a renewed interest in the setting up of PASS which is to be welcomed. PASS gives a local opportunity to support colleagues who are struggling; an opportunity to move beyond 'remedial' towards being the place where dental professionals discuss and explore issues, get support, and create a peer learning environment. A practical message from one of the projects was: 'Prevention is better than cure'. To be able to do this well other characteristics of PASS are important, for example to be confidential and non-judgemental, two most important practical messages. Together these are ingredients in providing the 'safe place' also noted as a practical message. Once practitioners trust that PASS is a safe place that is confidential and non-judgemental then the real magic can happen. This is the magic of support from a colleague who understands the struggles and pressures of dentistry and can support and give trusted advice.

Currently most PASS provide one to one mentoring/coaching. An interesting development is working with small groups. This could either be groups of professionals from the same practice or department or groups of individuals from different working environments. The link would be the issues that the group is working on. In these situations, the mentoring becomes a group activity led and facilitated by the 'core' mentor. The best group mentoring develops into co-mentoring within the group which escalates the learning for all. Inter-professional team mentoring is another development within PASS where mentoring for the whole team is facilitated by an experienced mentor. In these situations, the potential for reverse mentoring and co-mentoring become much more likely and desirable. The essential ingredient is the experienced mentor who is able to cross the boundaries of facilitator, coach, and tutor melding the process to the needs of the team.

As PASS develops its' role from remediation to embrace prevention the next step could be mentoring for excellence. These three phases are interlinked (Figure 6.1), and a dynamic relationship can be envisaged where the mentoring support oscillates between them.

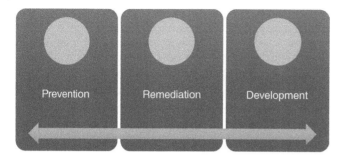

Figure 6.1 Phases for PASS.

Key take away messages: Support and advice for dental professionals by dental professionals can have an important and helpful impact on reducing or minimising performance difficulties. It can also provide a measure of prevention of performance difficulties escalating into major concerns. There could be a future role of mentoring for development and excellence using similar mechanisms and a model similar to PASS.

Health and Well-Being

Work by Rada and Johnson-Leong (2004) and Alexander (2001) showed that dentists live an average of 2.8 years longer than the general population which sounds like good news. Unfortunately, it seems dentists are also at greater risk of mental health issues, see Myers and Myers (2004), Puriene (2008). Research from other Countries indicates that this risk is not unique to the UK and that dentists across the world are prone to anxiety and depression, Rada and Johnson-Leong (2004), Puriene et al. (2008), Mathias (2005), Galan et al. (2014), Gorter (1998), Ahola and Hakanen (2007).

Ill health in dental professionals is well reported, with numerous studies into physical and mental health and addiction problems that can beset those working in dentistry, (Kay and Lowe 2008; Myers and Myers 2004). Dentists are notoriously a 'hard to reach' group when it comes to accessing healthcare because they can often be reluctant to seek treatment for their personal health problems. Thus it is imperative to find out more about how best to assist them on their road to recovery (excerpted from Brooks (2017, p. 16)). Linking back to the section on personal performance, early preventive mentoring supplied by a PASS could also act as a preventive for the onset of health problems.

There is extensive evidence to suggest that poor mental health can have detrimental effects on a person's overall physical health, social health, and quality of life. Hence the importance of maintaining good overall mental health. Not only is dentistry considered a highly stressful career but it is also perceived as more stressful compared to other occupations (Moore and Brodsgaard 2001; Myers and Myers 2004). All members of the dental team can be (and are) affected.

A study by Gill et al. (2008) postulated that mentoring relationships could have positive effects on the mental health of both mentees and mentors. 'The study suggests that a relatively inexpensive practice such as mentoring can help reduce anxiety among both senior and junior staff, and this could help organisations address the serious and costly workplace issues of anxiety and mental health'. A field experiment conducted by the team found that those who were part of the mentoring programme experienced lower levels of anxiety and a feeling that their job was more meaningful. These effects were however described as marginal. Anecdotally mentors in the dental profession have also reported that undertaking mentoring gives them a sense of value, giving back to others and being meaningful.

The study by Gill et al. was undertaken within the police force, however they state:

> 'While the study focused on high-stress roles in the public eye, we believe that the findings may also apply to other occupations that also have anxiety-provoking pressures'.

It would seem to be the case that dental professionals also operate in a high stress role in the public eye and that the findings do have relevance for dentistry.

Strengthening and building emotional resilience is important in being able to cope with vulnerability and what life throws at us. Burnout is a very real concern. Hakanen and Koivumaki (2014) state that burnout is grounded in pressure – emotional, cognitive, physical, and quantitative. This makes it difficult to pinpoint the exact causal factors for any one individual. Ahola and Hakanen (2007) found that burnout could trigger depression. Maslach and Jackson (1981) developed an inventory underpinning three key aspects of burnout: emotional exhaustion, depersonalisation (a cynical detached feeling towards patients), and a reduced sense of personal achievement. Gorter (2000) suggests that there is a continuum with engagement at one extreme and burnout at the other, respectively characterised by energy (versus exhaustion), involvement (versus cynicism), and efficacy (versus inefficacy) (p. 38).

Chipchase et al. (2017) built on Maslach's work on burnout and concluded that:

> Dentists' anxiety in clinical situations does affect the way that dentists work clinically, as assessed using the newly designed and validated Dentists' Anxieties in Clinical Situation Scale (DACSS). This anxiety is associated with measures of burnout and decision-making style.

In addition, they established that burnout can impact a dentist's work with: 'effects on decision making; modifying treatment plans, referring-on, effects on treatment given, changes to procedures and interpersonal interactions and effects on style of decision –making'.

The BDA has undertaken several surveys and research into the health of dental professionals (Larbie et al. 2017). Mentoring was given as one of the top three suggestions from interviewees of the 2017 survey for the best ways to prevent burnout and ill health

Research by Gill et al. (2018) suggest that mentoring programmes can have a positive impact on both mentees' and mentors' mental health. They found that 'mentoring relationships provide a unique context for mentors to discuss and normalise their concerns, to share ideas for managing anxieties, and to find more meaning in their work'.

An important aspect of health and well-being is resilience. Whilst psychological resilience can be difficult to conceptualise and define, it is generally accepted as the ability to recover from significant stress or adversity. Building our resilience is a protective and preventive measure and for dental professionals who work in a high stress environment optimum resilience is a must rather than a nice extra. There are many books on resilience and some excellent courses. Linda Graham (2015) introduces the five C's or resilient coping:

1) **Calm**: You can stay calm in a crisis.
2) **Clarity**: You can see clearly what's happening as well as your internal response to what's happening; you can see what needs to happen next; and you can see possibilities from different perspectives that will enhance your ability to respond flexibly.
3) **Connection:** You can reach out for help as needed; you can learn from others how to be resilient; and you can connect to resources that greatly expand your options.
4) **Competence**: You can call on skills and competencies that you have learned through previous experience (or that you learn) to act quickly and effectively.
5) **Courage**: You can strengthen your faith to persevere in your actions until you come to resolution or acceptance of the difficulty.

It seems appropriate at the time of writing (summer 2020) to add a few words about the impact the COVID-19 pandemic has had on the health and wellbeing issues raised in the coaching and mentoring field. Professionally-trained mentors and coaches cover emotional intelligence in their training, notably the ability to be empathetic, compassionate, and receptive to discussing strong emotions.

The pandemic has raised issues of anxiety, uncertainty, loss of income, loss of career, dental businesses, and tragically, loss of family members, friends, and colleagues.

Bereavement counselling is a specialist area of practise and yet, because mentors and coaches are approachable and offer a listening ear, and have the ability to talk through challenging issues and signpost to other services as needed, mentors are finding themselves supporting clients in this way.

The one glimmer of good news is that people are showing signs of being more willing to talk about matters that touch on their own health and wellbeing. Health professionals are, traditionally, notoriously reluctant to talk about their feelings and yet the COVID-19 situation has made the discussions of our fears and feelings much more commonplace.

Mentors have an important role to play in this 'normalising' process, as they can offer a different dimension: everyday conversations that are also profound and supportive in challenging times.

Key Take Away Messages

The mentoring relationship can have a positive impact on the mental health, well-being, and resilience of both mentee and mentor. Mentoring could increase resilience and protect against burnout.

Communication

A theme present in several case studies across the different categories was the importance of communication. Communication is at the centre of the mentoring relationship. Case study 12 is a good example of a model that can be integrated into the dental practice. Case study 11 introduces coaching cards, an interesting way to begin a deeper level of communication. A really good mentor will have excellent communication, both verbal and non-verbal. Communication is so much more than talking. The best partnerships are those where the mentor is skilled in listening, asking great questions and then listening again. Deep listening is listening that really hears what the mentee is saying both verbally and non-verbally. It hears what is conveyed and what is not conveyed. It hears emotions, beliefs, and values. People communicate with words, gestures, expression, movements of their bodies and silence. A skilled mentor picks up on all these forms of communication. Sometimes listening is the greatest gift that the mentor can bring to the relationship.

For those case studies supporting dental professionals in difficulty through PASS, an understanding of the situations that others have found challenging is important: 'Support and Advice group run by dentists for dentists'; 'You are not alone'; 'To let all those who need it know that there are others going through the same as them and that there are people to share and support them'; 'Modern dentistry is becoming ever more stressful as a result of a number of factors and cultural environment'. Mentoring improves communication skills and can convey a lasting legacy for both mentors and mentees in having better conversations with those around them, including, and importantly patients.

Sullivan and Decker (2009) note that the goal of communication is: 'to approach, as closely as possible, a common understanding of the message sent, and the one received'. They confirm the two-way nature of communication. It is not to tell, but to send and receive.

Interestingly they suggest a variety of factors that influence communication, these are:

- Past conditioning
- The present situation
- Each person's purpose in the communication
- Each person's attitudes towards self, the topic, and each other.

These factors will influence the communication that takes place during the mentor/mentee relationship, for example, in the following ways:

- If the mentee has previously had good experiences of mentoring they will be far more receptive to the relationship than someone who has not.
- If the present situation is that mentoring is being provided because of concerns with poor performance and participation in the relationship has been mandated by a third party, the mentee may see the intervention as punitive and something they have been told to take part in. They may be resistant to engaging.
- If the mentor believes that their purpose is to judge and direct their mentee, then the relationship will be less fruitful.
- If the mentor finds it difficult to work with their mentee because the topic is one they are uncomfortable with then the relationship is more likely to fail.

The experienced mentor is aware of these factors and the extent to which each may influence their relationship with a specific mentee. Awareness is a step towards controlling the influence a factor has.

Key Take Away Messages

Communication is the bed rock of the mentoring relationship and conversation. Whilst clinicians are generally competent communicators they should take time to explore the dimensions of communication to improve their understanding and competence. Deep listening is the core of mentoring.

Mentoring and Coaching as Regular and Every Day

Another important theme that crossed case studies was that mentoring should become so embedded within dentistry that it becomes a regular habit, present everywhere for everyone and not seen as something that should be reserved for the domain of poor performance and remediation. Mentoring is such a powerful relationship and the rewards are so great that everyone should enjoy the benefits.

There will always be a place for experienced and specially trained mentors to work in the fields of remediation and career development. However much more could be available for personal development, and personal development never stops. Building on this theme there was a recognition that mentoring should be available for all members of the dental team and should not only be considered with regard to dentists. Currently PASS generally provides mentoring for dentists, which neglects the majority of dental professionals. If we are to provide the most effective healthcare to patients, mentoring schemes should be made available to the whole team throughout their careers.

Key Take Away Messages

Mentoring is a state of being more than it is of doing. It should be part of everyday conversation. All dental professionals should have access to mentoring.

Supportive Culture for Coaching and Mentoring

A theme of developing a more empathic and supportive culture for each other within dentistry was evident. A shift of emphasis from punitive to developmental approaches when dealing with performance issues was clearly considered to be desirable. Such a change of emphasis could impact on levels of stress and anxiety for practitioners who are identified as struggling and requiring support. A knock on effect of a kinder, more humanistic shift would be enhanced patient care as practitioners sought support at a much earlier stage. It is likely that ill health episodes experienced by individuals could also be reduced.

Most practices and departments are comprised of a relatively small number of individuals who work together closely. Whilst it is obviously important to place patient care and clinical interventions as the priority offering in dentistry, for that to happen people need to feel supported and valued. Time needs to be invested in building a solid team that looks out for one another, that knows the pressures and anxieties that each bring to the practice.

What happens away from the practice underpins what happens within the practice. It is rare for any individual to completely leave non-work concerns at home (or vice versa); consequently, compassionate management, and leadership gets the best from all members of the team. Individuals who feel empowered to share concerns are far more likely to talk to their colleagues at an early stage when concerns can be resolved comparatively easily. Practices that embrace mentoring are more likely to develop an overarching supportive culture.

Key Take Away Messages

People need to feel valued, supported, and that they matter. Time taken to team build and mentor brings dividends in productivity of individuals and a willingness to invest themselves in the practice. Mentoring makes good business sense.

Share and Enjoy

The people who shared their case studies all felt that there was potential for the transference of ideas used in dentistry to other fields both within and outside of health services. Tools and models used primarily by mentors and coaches can be used more generically to underpin personal development plans and appraisal systems in many other areas of work. For example, the use of evaluation of reflective writing has wide application within and outside healthcare. The benefits of mentoring apply throughout learning and should be employed in all workplaces. Mentoring schemes used during the early years of the dental professional could be replicated to benefit younger and less experienced people in most professions and forms of employment.

Larbie et al. (2017) suggest that promoting connectivity within the profession can grow support networks that help combat isolation and build resilience. Peer mentoring networks are one such mechanism. The study also noted that there are particular critical points during a dentist's career where such support can be of especial value; one example being the transition from trainee to independent practitioner, see case studies eight and nine. Another transition can be the move from Associate to Principal or on achieving specialist or consultant status.

Mentoring programmes can be scaled up or down depending on the size of an organisation, whether a small dental practice, a large corporate body, a community service or a hospital department. The frameworks described within the case studies can be adapted for personal development and leadership in any organisational structure. Ultimately such programmes are beneficial to dental professionals and patient care.

Key Take Away Messages

Copy with pride (while acknowledging and crediting where the idea came from). Mentoring can be particularly beneficial at transition points in our careers.

Integrating Mentoring into Structures and Systems

The Whole Professional Career

This topic links well with the early years' case studies, the prevention/minimisation of problems and the promotion of excellence. If mentoring can be introduced early into an individual's training and career, there is a real prospect that it will become embedded into their routine practice which sets the direction towards mentoring throughout their whole career.

A number of dental schools and other training establishments have introduced mentoring schemes for their undergraduate dental professionals and trainees. It is also important that, once qualified, dental professionals continue to engage in mentoring. In the early years post qualification learning continues at a fast pace and without guidance it can be difficult to grow professionally and develop appropriate decision making. Foundation and vocational training schemes offer the support of educational supervisors most of whom have been trained in mentoring skills. Once that year has been completed young dentists find themselves in truly independent practice and this can be a daunting time. It is a crucial time for mentoring to continue to be a regular feature in any young dentist's practice.

Several of the case studies described in Chapter 5 are aimed at embedding mentoring into the early years of a dental professional's career, from dental school to independent practice via foundation/vocational training. The hope is that mentoring becomes a habit that is valued and continued throughout the career.

Mentoring, both as experienced by the mentor and the mentee is beyond a value metric, it pervades all aspects of the profession and practice of dentistry. It has value in minimising poor performance, value in improved patient care, engagement, and co-operation, practice management, team dynamics, and value in shifting good to excellent performance.

The value is also in greater emotional payback. Perhaps this is because of the non-judgemental sharing and the trust that develops between mentor and mentee. It is a therapeutic relationship – without being a 'therapy' – that can have a huge positive impact on the individuals directly involved but also those around them, who may not be directly mentored but benefit from the results of mentoring.

It is possible to be both a mentor and be mentored, in fact that is perhaps the most beneficial – a mentoring matrix. At all stages of the professional career mentoring is of benefit. As noted in one of the projects: 'Mentoring is just the way you become, it shouldn't be forced or false. It is positive for everyone involved and helps all sides develop personally and professionally'. Mentoring is just the way you become, such a great sentiment. Mentoring moves from something you do to something you are.

Schrubbe (2009), discussing the use of mentoring support for students, commends it as a tool supporting professional growth and development as well as academic success.

Gagliardi and Wright (2010) evaluated a surgical skills mentorship programme in Canada. They found that the mentoring relationship impacted on knowledge and attitudes in a positive manner and that clinical outcomes of the mentees was also improved. In addition, the relationship benefits flowed both ways enhancing self-reflection and the sharing of knowledge and expertise between mentors and mentees. The Canadian programme also found that mentoring between known colleagues, and which took place within the mentee's clinical environment, were seen as being particularly valuable. There is a transferable message here for mentoring between educational supervisors and foundation/vocational trainees in dentistry.

Key Take Away Messages

Start good mentoring habits early and keep them up.

Organisational Culture

Organisational culture is a fascinating topic. It defines the intrinsic nature of an organisation, regardless of size. The culture is comprised of a number of aspects including values, beliefs, how people work with each other, how decisions are made and how work is done. Culture within an organisation has a history and often survives changes in management. This is a feature that many a new principal has found to their cost when taking over a practice where the culture is already set.

In the Forton Coaching and Mentoring model, 'culture' is defined as the combination of the individual's inner thoughts, beliefs, and values – as enacted in their words and deeds

– and the group or team's thoughts, beliefs, and values enacted in expected patterns of speech and behaviour. This 'whole system' approach is based on the work of Wilber (1996) and will vary from organisation to organisation, and even department to department. Think of the culture in a dental practice compared to, say, a supermarket; or compare the culture of a sales department to a finance team.

An understanding of a specific culture is important when trying to make changes. Those changes that are in line with the culture will be easier to make and those that are out of kilter with the culture will be very difficult and unlikely to succeed. When considering the introduction of mentoring to an organisation for the first time, the existing culture could make that introduction fairly easy, or it could make it impossible. Good ideas can fail if the organisational culture does not support them.

Myth Busting

So much is written about mentoring and coaching. Over the years, myths have built up and most of them are negative, if you listen to the myths you could be put off. If that is the case it would be a great loss, to you, and to the people around you. This short section looks at some of the more common myths and attempts to debunk them.

'Deskilling'

The myth to be busted: Mentoring skills are only to be used in formal mentoring situations. So if you do not undertake formal mentoring relatively frequently you will deskill.

Use it or lose it – I'm sure you have heard that phrase a few times. It probably has quite a bit of truth in it, but does it apply to mentoring? Mentoring is a combination of experience to share and supporting the mentee to 'do it for themselves'. The experience a mentor has to share may change over time, the most extreme example is post retirement from the profession, this is particularly the case for clinical skills. Dentistry and the health service changes rapidly and within a relatively short time an individual may feel out of touch and out of date. However, the skills of coaching, which do not rely on specific or detailed know-how, do not date in the same way. This means that, with continued development a mentor can transition to a coach and continue to apply their valuable skills. There is also the possibility of training as a supervisor for mentors.

What about the skills of supporting a mentee, can those become rusty if not used? Yes, they could. Let us refresh what those skills are. Listening, asking questions, being present. These skills are transferable to any and every setting a dental professional finds themselves in. Whether they are working clinically or non-clinically the skills of supporting can be used and should be used.

In short, the experience and skills a mentor has to offer are unlikely to become rusty, if applied daily and kept updated. Once acquired mentoring skills become a way of interaction with others, a way of having better conversations with everyone, work, home or play. In this way, the mentor is unlikely to become deskilled. Of course, it is important to keep up CPD in mentoring skills, this is a professional expectation.

Anyone Can Mentor

The myth to be busted: All dental professionals can automatically mentor without additional training.

The notion that anyone can mentor rather devalues the skill of mentoring and the skills mentors need to acquire. Not every dental professional can mentor well, not everyone is cut out for it and not everyone demonstrates the skills proficiently enough to be a good mentor, although all can improve. Most dental professionals who have a skill or experience of sufficient depth to be useful to share with another can learn the skills needed to be a mentor. It's important to note that the skills do need to be learnt, even those who are 'naturals' can hone and improve their ability with training. With advanced training good mentors can become excellent mentors.

Age – 'reverse mentoring'

The myth to be busted: Mentoring is a one-way transaction – older to younger. If someone has experience that you would like to acquire and they have the skills to support your learning, listen to them!

Age is such a strange phenomenon. When you are young, you think you know everything, as you get older you realise you know nothing!!! We used to joke about asking a seven-year old to show us how to work the video player (how technology shows our age). Today it's more about using social media, understanding the digital revolution and connecting with young people. Humour apart, it can seem counter intuitive to be mentored by someone younger than yourself. However, experience and skill are not necessarily a factor of age. The statement that the older you are the more experienced and skilful you are does not always hold true. It depends on the skill.

In this technological age it is common for younger members of the profession to have skills that older members either do not have or are less proficient in. Examples are IT, digital technology, social platforms, new materials – the list is a long one. A great example of reverse mentoring can be found in the relationship between Educational Supervisor and Foundation/Vocational Trainee. In most instances the trainee is acquiring knowledge and skill in working in the real world of dentistry, honing their clinical skills, learning what it takes to run a practice, understanding team working and a 101 other skills.

However, it's not a one-way street, the trainee can also pass on knowledge to the supervisor in areas of digital technology, up to the minute techniques, new materials that they have experienced at dental school. Let us also not forget that trainees are generally excited about working in dentistry, they have enthusiasm and a desire to serve patients that can be refreshing for those who qualified a few years ago.

When older, more experienced people are open to innovative ideas and new ways of doing old things from younger people, the combination of novelty is balanced with experience; new ideas can evolve from the old. Helping to see colleagues through their eyes builds empathy and trust, quickly. In today's highly digital age, reverse mentoring is vital.

Inter-professional Mentoring

The myth to be busted: You must only choose a mentor from the same professional group as yourself.

As described throughout the book, mentoring has two major components; skill or experience that is of value to another and the skills to support another. When that is understood it becomes a short jump to realise that a professional colleague from any of the professional groups in dentistry may have a skill or experience that would be of value to someone from another professional group. In this way a dental nurse who has experience of project management, or a dental therapist who has trained in special care dentistry, or a clinical dental technician who has skills in patient management could mentor a colleague from a different professional group who wishes to deepen their own skills in that particular area. The important consideration is whether the mentor has the supporting skills and do they have a particular experience or skill that the mentee wishes to acquire. The specific professional group is not an important criterion.

Holt and Ladwa (2010), stress both the value of mentor training and how all members of the dental team might contribute to the mentoring role.

The aim of this study was to examine whether newly qualified healthcare staff can be supported in their journey to become a practitioner using an inter-professional framework to mentoring. The study involved the mentoring of newly qualified doctors (pre-registration house officers – PRHOs) by senior nurses for the first six months of their clinical practice. The findings from this study show that mentoring using an inter-professional method is a viable approach to supporting professionals, particularly during the early stages of their professional lives and in the current health service climate. Inter-professional mentoring was perceived as a means for supporting the personal and professional development of newcomers as well as the professional development of the mentors. In the author's personal experience they received excellent mentoring from a senior dental nurse when they first began to practice, fresh out of dental school. Her experiences of the clinic, the patients, policies, and processes was invaluable.

Reflection Is Not Measurable; Therefore, Not Worthwhile

Myth to be busted: Reflection is impossible to measure.

Reflection is a seriously underutilised learning style and skill. It's not that dental professionals do not reflect; they do. However, it is rare for reflection to be used to its maximum potential. If asked, most dental professionals would say they reflect, although most are unaware of models of reflection and few write their reflections down. Even then, it is a powerful way of learning. Reflection is learning from personal experience, it is practical. Reflection most commonly comes after an action. The action could be undertaken for a clinical procedure, or a conversation, or a lecture, or following an audit, or following a complaint. Reflection can also take place whilst the action is being undertaken, known as 'in action' although as noted above most commonly the reflection takes place after the action, known as 'on action'. It can seem as if reflection is undervalued, why is this? Perhaps because it is less easy to translate reflection into business potential. Perhaps because time taken to think is not seen as productive time. Dental professionals generally identify most often as activists when considering the Honey and Mumford learning styles (1982), they like to do practical things. Activists may view reflection as time wasted. However, time taken to reflect on why an action either was less successful or more successful can improve the chances of either errors not being repeated or successes becoming more frequent. Fewer errors and more successes directly translate into business success which has an economic value.

Reflection is often a skill that mentors can support mentees to improve upon. A difficulty can be that individuals are not sure how to evaluate and really use their own reflections. Most dental professionals are good at describing events, but this is not reflection and reflection is personal. The case study in Chapter 5 outlines a method via which reflective writing can be measured and evaluated. This makes it an excellent tool for feedback. Just because reflection and reflective writing in particular is a qualitative instrument does not mean it cannot be measured and evaluated.

Failure Is Failure – Or Is It an Opportunity to Learn and Improve?

Myth to be busted: Failure is a bad thing and must be avoided, or forgotten as quickly as possible.

Failure is a difficult concept and can be viewed as a taboo subject. It has negative connotations in many areas of life, 'no one wants to be labelled a failure'. Yet, failure is a critical part of success. It is rare for a person to successfully complete a task the first time they attempt it.

This begins early. Babies learning to walk and talk rarely begin with a word perfect speech or being able to walk without falling over, indeed standing is quite the feat at first. I can remember how long it took me to ride a bike without wobbling all over the place and falling off. As a dental student I demolished many a plastic tooth before I acquired the skill to cut cavities. Failure is part of success, we fail, we learn, we fail again, we learn more. We repeat and repeat and finally, success. Each failure teaches a lesson, each failure builds upon the previous one and we get better. Failure as the forerunner of success is built into our very DNA. Nature has created many a blind alley along the path of evolution.

Making an error is not the issue, it's failing to learn from that error so that the chance of the same error occurring again is minimised. Failing to learn from failure is the real problem. The failure is not that an error was made, the failure is that the opportunity to learn and improve was missed. Mentors are key to supporting colleagues turn failures into opportunities to learn and improve. Failure can be particularly difficult for those who have not experienced it. For example, dental students and young dentists who are academically high fliers may find their first failure devastating. Those who have experienced failure early on have learnt greater resilience and are less affected by it. There is no success without failure.

No Time to Mentor

Myth to be busted: I have no time to mentor – yes you do. Do not do, be.

Mentoring is just another thing to fit into an already packed working day. Whilst it is true that there are times when mentoring requires specific time to be allocated, it is by no means always the case. The skills required for mentoring, once acquired become a way of being, a way of having better conversations with everyone. Doing is replaced by being. It can be as easy as shifting the way questions are asked. Asking questions with curiosity often produces more value and takes no longer in time. Just a little practice.

A Note for Covid-19

At the time of writing the COVID-19 pandemic has had a sudden, rapid, and profound impact on the delivery of dental services and dental professionals in the UK and across the globe. It is not clear whether the changes to delivery are longer term, or indeed permanent (the 'new normal'), it is too soon to tell. Nonetheless, what is clear is that mentoring and coaching has a number of immediate roles to play:

- Dental service delivery: supporting dental professionals to adapt to sudden change, and helping them support their colleagues and team members in turn.
- Dental business: as well as signposting to financial counselling, career, and other business support services, being an approachable and supportive ear at times of severe pressure on practice owners and associates, enabling them to make the best possible business decisions in the circumstances.
- Dental education and training: supporting the profession to adapt its training methods and approaches, to maintain high standards.
- Dental careers: helping people discover what options they have within the profession and to support those who are re-thinking their career options and decisions, in the light of the pandemic.
- Health and wellbeing: using their skills both to hold empathetic and compassionate conversations at times of great anxiety and uncertainty, and to take a signposting role, so that dental professionals get access to the best possible specialist services and information.
- Redeployment of dental professionals: supporting the many dental professionals who answered the call for redeployment and worked in a number of non-dental capacities, including front line care of Covid-19 patients.

Many dental coach/mentors have stepped up to the plate to support colleagues, often in a pro bono capacity.

Dental professionals, in our experience, have more resilience, skills, and abilities than they know. Mentors have the skills to bring these resources, and resourcefulness, out in people. It's not just that they have the skills to help people discover ways out of the maze, it is that having a clear set of professional values and skills help create an environment for calm and clear decision-making.

Conclusion

Mentoring and coaching in the dental profession is a maturing practise and has already shown its value to individuals and organisations. Whilst practical and attitudinal barriers still remain, its benefits are clear: reducing stress and burnout, improving resilience, supporting professionals throughout their career journeys and helping them make the right choices at critical career moments. Mentoring is more than fixing poor performance, putting right complaints or dealing with patient failures; it's about encouraging excellence and supporting the structural and technological changes in the profession now, and in the months and years ahead.

Mentoring and coaching is not just about one-to-one conversations, it reaches into reflective practise, and can be a team or group activity. However, it demands leadership from the profession: where we are reflective professionals ourselves, modelling the behaviours we expect of others. It means being more coach-like as leaders, not just mentoring in formal settings.

Our maturity gives us the chance to interact with other health professions on an equal footing, where coaching, and mentoring is increasingly being offered, adapted, and explored to support those professions, and healthcare professionals allied to medicine. We can both learn from other professional coaches and mentors, through the range of associations, conferences and research activities, and give back from our own experience. We see the kind of coaching and mentoring practised in the dental profession as invaluable to other technical and professional job roles and to coaches and mentors working in other highly regulated fields.

It's also a great time to explore the opportunities afforded by the 'Virtual Revolution' of coaching at a distance: thus cutting out travel, accommodation, and time costs. Of experimenting with 'reverse mentoring', so that experienced dental professionals benefit from the digital generations and the benefits available to patients and professionals alike from these new technologies. Mentoring and coaching are about performance improvement and re-skilling, not de-skilling. This means that, far from pursuing traditional dentistry options for too long, career options for dental professionals can expand into new and exciting fields.

All of this requires further support from the profession: we need a supportive culture within which mentoring and coaching can thrive. This requires the removal of attitudinal barriers, where 'performance conversations' aren't a synonym for punishment, but are truly opportunities to improve and excel. This needs to come through national, regional, and local policies; through the corporate bodies, the indemnity providers and the specialist societies. The BDA has led the way in this regard, already hosting two international conferences for mentoring and coaching at its London offices. While the climate at the time of writing prevents largely in-person conferences, we hope that the situation soon permits us to reconvene in person. Of course, as we write this, there is a growing appetite for online conferences as a reasonable alternative.

But coaching and mentoring does not depend on policy-making alone. It is through people that we change culture and we look forward to watching modern mentoring become the norm across the dental profession.

We hope that the case studies, and the issues they raise, give you pause for thought about introducing mentoring and coaching into your organisation; whether to address complaints; develop people's capabilities, or to make excellence a habit for all. We encourage you to adapt the ideas here to bring coaching and mentoring into your workplace; reflect on your own skillset as a mentor or coach, keep developing, and applying your skills so that everyone benefits.

References

Ahola, K. and Hakanen, J. (2007). Job strain, burnout, and depressive symptoms: a prospective study among dentists. *Journal of Affective Disorders* 104 (1–3): 103–110.

Alexander, R.E. (2001). Stress-related suicide by dentists and other health care workers: fact or folklore? *Journal of the American Dental Association* 132 (6): 786–794.

Brooks, J.A. (2017). *How to Survive Dental Performance Difficulties.* Wiley Blackwell. ISBN: 978-1-119-25561-1.

Chipchase, S.Y., Chapman, H.R., and Bretherton, R. (2017). A study to explore if dentists' anxiety affects their clinical decision-making. *British Dental Journal* 222 (4): 277–290.

EMCC Position Paper on the European Skills Agenda, 22 July 2020. Brussels

Forton. (2020), https://thefortongroup.com/images/downloads/2017materials/ FortonCaseStudies.pdf" https://thefortongroup.com/images/downloads/2017materials/ FortonCaseStudies.pdf

Gagliardi, A.R. and Wright, F.C. (2010). Exploratory evaluation of surgical skills mentorship program design and outcomes. *Journal of Continuing Education in the Health Professions* 30: 51–56.

Galán, F., Ríos-Santos, J.V., Polo, J. et al. (2014). Burnout, depression and suicidal ideation in dental students. *Medicina Oral, Patología Oral y Cirugía Bucal* 19 (3): 206–211.

Gill, M., Roulet, T., and Kerridge, S. (2018). Mentoring for mental health: a mixed-method study of the benefits of formal mentoring programmes in the English police force. *Journal of Vocational Behavior* 108: 201–213. https://doi.org/10.1016/j.jvb.2018.08.005.

Golman, D., Boyatzis, R., and McKee, A. (2002). *The New Leaders: Transforming the Art of Leadership in to the Science of Results.* Little, Brown.

Gorter, R. (2000). Burnout and health among Dutch dentists. *European Journal of Oral Sciences* 108 (4): 261–267.

Gorter, R.C., Albrecht, G., Hoogstraten, J. et al. (1998). Work place characteristics, work stress and burnout among Dutch dentists. *European Journal of Oral Sciences* 106: 999–1005.

Graham, L. (2015). *Bouncing Back: Rewiring Your Brain for Maximum Resilience and Well-Being,* Kindle. New World Library.

Hakanen, J. and Koivumaki, J. (2014). Engaged or exhausted – how does it affect dentists' clinical productivity? *Burnout Research* 1: 12–18.

Holt, V.P. and Ladwa, R. (2010). Developing a mentoring culture in dentistry. Making a difference in a changing world. *Primary Dental Care* 17: 93–98.

Honey, P. and Mumford, A. (1982). *Manual of Learning Styles.* London: P. Honey.

Kay, E.J. and Lowe, J.C. (2008). A survey of stress levels, self-perceived health and health-related behaviours of UK dental practitioners in 2005. *British Dental Journal* 204: E19. 56.

Larbie, J., Kemp, M., Whitehead, P., (2017). The mental health and well-being of UK Dentists: A qualitative survey. BDA Research Paper. *British Dental Association*

Maslach, C. and Jackson, S.E. (1981). The measurement of experienced burnout. *Journal of Occupational Behaviour* 2: 99–113.

Mathias, S., Koeber, A., Fadavi, S., and Punwani, I. (2005). Specialty and sex as predictors of depression in dentists. *The Journal of the American Dental Association* 136 (10): 1388–1395.

Moore, R. and Brodsgaard, I. (2001). Dentists' perceived stress and its relation to perceptions about anxious patients. *Community Dental and Oral Epidemiology* 29 (1): 73–80.

Myers and Myers (2004). 'It's difficult being a dentist': stress and health in the general dental practitioner. *British Dental Journal* 197: 89–93.

Puriene, A., Aleksejuiene, J., Petrauskiene, J. et al. (2008). Self-perceived mental health and job satisfaction among Lithuanian dentists. *Industrial Health* 46: 247–252.

Rada, R.E. and Johnson-Leong, C. (2004). Stress, burnout, anxiety and depression among dentists. *Journal of the American Dental Association* 135 (6): 788–794.

Schrubbe, K.F. (2009). Mentorship: a critical component for professional growth and academic success. *Journal of Dental Education* 68 (3): 324–328.

Soumya, B.G. and Ramachandra, S.S. (2011). Haptics application in dentistry: is the time poised yet? *Dental Hypotheses* 2: 9–15. https://doi.org/10.5436/j.dehy.2011.2.00019, https://www.researchgate.net/publication/49611327_Haptics_Application_in_Dentistry_Is_the_Time_Poised_Yet (accessed 10 August 2020).

Sullivan, E.S. and Decker, P.J. (2009). *Effective Leadership and Management in Nursing*, 7e. Upper Saddle River, NJ: Pearson Prentice Hall.

Wilber, K. (1996). *A Brief History of Everything*. Shambhala Publications.

Glossary of Terms – Organisations and Other Descriptors

Organisations

British Dental Association (BDA) The British Dental Association is the professional association and registered trade union organisation for dentists in the United Kingdom. Its stated mission is to 'promote the interests of members, advance the science, arts and ethics of dentistry and improve the nation's oral health'.

Care Quality Commission (CQC) The Care Quality Commission is an executive non-departmental public body of the Department of Health and Social Care of the United Kingdom. It was established in 2009 to regulate and inspect health and social care services in England.

Chartered Institute of Personnel and Development (CIPD) A professional association for human resource management professionals.

Chartered Management Institute (CMI) The Chartered Management Institute is a professional institution for management based in the United Kingdom.

Committee of Postgraduate Dental Deans and Directors (COPDEND) A committee of all Postgraduate Dental Deans and Directors in the UK. It oversees postgraduate training for dentists; European Economic Area and overseas dentists and workforce development.

Community Dental Service (CDS) Community Dental Services provide treatment for people who may not otherwise seek or receive dental care, such as people with learning disabilities, elderly housebound people, people with mental or physical health problems or other disabling conditions which prevent them from visiting a general dental practitioner.

Deaneries Postgraduate medical and dental training is available for all doctors and dentists in England. The teams that do this work in HEE, are now part of local teams. They may also be referred to as Post Graduate Medical and Dental Education or healthcare education (HET) teams.

Dental Complaints Service (DCS) The Dental Complaints Service (DCS) is a team of trained advisers whose aim to help private dental patients and professionals settle complaints about private dental care fairly and efficiently. Funded by the GDC, the DCS provides a free and impartial service to mediate between patient and professional.

Practical Applications of Coaching and Mentoring in Dentistry, First Edition.
Janine Brooks and Helen Caton-Hughes.
© 2021 John Wiley & Sons Ltd. Published 2021 by John Wiley & Sons Ltd.

Dentists' Health Support Trust (DHST) The Dentists' Health Support Trust offers dentists in difficulty an opportunity to remedy their problems, get their life back on track and, where possible, back into practice. The Trust provides a number of services including: responding to enquiries, which may lead to intervention, assessments, and treatment pathways followed by ongoing monitoring and support. This support is extended to families and colleagues of the dental professional in difficulty.

Department of Health and Social Care (DHSC) Supports ministers in leading the nation's health and social care to help people live more independent, healthier lives for longer. DHSC is a ministerial department, supported by 29 agencies and public bodies. Prior to 2018 known as Department of Health.

European Mentoring and Coaching Council (EMCC) The European Mentoring and Coaching Council provides coaching and mentoring professional accreditation, as well as support and guidance to the coaching and mentoring profession and for its members.

General Dental Council (GDC) The General Dental Council is the UK-wide statutory regulator of members of the dental team. Its primary purpose is to protect patient safety and maintain public confidence in dental services. To achieve this, the Council registers qualified dental professionals, set standards for the dental team, investigates complaints about dental professionals' fitness to practise, and works to ensure the quality of dental education.

Health Board (HB) There are 14 regional NHS Boards in Scotland which are responsible for the protection and the improvement of their population's health and for the delivery of frontline healthcare services.

There are seven NHS Health Boards in Wales which plan, secure and deliver health-care services in their areas.

Health Education England (HEE) Health Education England is an executive non-departmental public body of the Department of Health and Social Care. Their function is to provide national leadership and coordination for the education and training within the health and public health workforce within England. It has been operational since June 2012.

Healthcare Education Team (HET) See Deanery above.

Healthwatch England (HWE) Healthwatch England is the independent national champion for people who use health and social care services. There is a local Healthwatch in every area of England.

Institute of Dentistry (IoD) Institute of Dentistry is one of the six institutes of Barts and the London School of Medicine and Dentistry (SMD), Queen Mary University of London (QMUL).

Institute of Leadership and Management (ILM) The Institute of Leadership & Management is a professional membership body for leaders and managers.

International Coach Federation (ICF) The International Coach Federation is a non-profit organisation dedicated to professional coaching. As of July 2020, ICF has approximately 41 500 members in 147 countries and territories.

Local Area Team (LAT) NHS England regional teams. There are seven regions in England who support local systems to provide more joined up and sustainable care for patients. Regional teams are responsible for the quality, financial and operational performance of all NHS organisations in their region, they draw on the expertise and support of the corporate teams to improve services for patients and support local transformation.

Local Dental Committee (LDC) Local Dental Committees exist throughout the UK. They are the democratically elected representative body for primary care NHS dentists at the local level. They have existed since the creation of the National Health Service to support and represent dentists and to help plan services in local areas.

Local Dental Network (LDN) Cover the whole dental pathway across primary, secondary and community care as well as out of hours services. They play a key role in supporting the development of quality measures for dental primary and secondary care. They work closely with local authorities and Public Health England to deliver and develop cohesive oral health strategies and associated commissioning plans.

National Health Service (NHS) The National Health Service is the umbrella term for the publicly-funded healthcare systems of the UK. Since 1948 it has been funded out of general taxation.

National Institute for Clinical Excellence (NICE) The National Institute for Clinical Excellence provides national guidance and advice to improve health and social care.

NHS Business Service Authority (NHSBSA) The NHS Business Services Authority is an Arm's Length Body of the Department of Health and Social Care. The Authority manage over £35 billion of NHS spend annually delivering a range of national services to NHS organisations, NHS contractors, patients and the public.

NHS England (NHSE) NHS England leads the National Health Service (NHS) in England.

Performance Advisory Group (PAG) NHS England has established Performance Advisory Groups and Performers Lists Decision Panels within local teams in order to support its responsibility in managing the performance of primary care performers. The PAG's role is to consider concerns about a named individual, who is either included on the Performers List, has a prescribed connection to NHS England, or is a Pharmacist, and determine the most appropriate course of action. It can instruct an investigation where it considers it appropriate and it can agree voluntary undertakings with a performer when low level concerns have been identified and the performer accepts this to be the case.

Performers List Decision Panel (PLDP) The primary role of the PLDP is to make decisions under the Performers Lists Regulations. This does not prevent the PLDP from taking any action that the PAG can take.

Postgraduate Medical and Dental Training (PMDT) The teams that do this work in HEE. They used to be deaneries, and are now part of local teams. They may also be referred to as the PGMDE or HET teams.

Practitioner Advice and Support Scheme (PASS) PASS was first developed in the 1990s with the first scheme being in Lancashire. It was first designed for those dentists in difficulty to be supported or mentored by experienced colleagues within the same region where they worked and its intention has remained broadly the same. In most situations it is coordinated and facilitated by Local Dental Committees (LDC). The ambition of a PASS is to be able to rehabilitate the dentist in difficulty such that they can continue in practice with their confidence restored and able to further contribute in an effective way within the profession.

Practitioner Performance Advice (PPA) Provide impartial advice to healthcare organisations in England, Wales and Northern Ireland to effectively manage and resolve concerns raised about the practice of individual practitioners. Formerly the National Clinical Assessment Service, (NCAS) established in 2001, now a service delivered by NHS Resolution under the common purpose, to provide expertise to the NHS on resolving concerns fairly, share from learning for improvement and preserve resources for patient care.

Public Health England (PHE) Protects and improves the nation's health and wellbeing, and reduces health inequalities. PHE is an executive agency, sponsored by the Department of Health and Social Care. A new National Institute for Health Protection (NIHP) took on the responsibilities of Public Health England, NHS Test and Trace and the analytical team from the Joint Biosecurity Centre (JBC) from Autumn 2020.

Qualifications Curriculum Authority (QCA) The Qualifications Curriculum Authority leads developments in management courses, curriculum, assessments, examinations, and qualifications.

Regulation of Dental Services Programme Board (RDSPB) A group formed of organisations with a role and responsibility for setting, managing and regulating how dental care is provided in England. It aims to jointly ensure that patients receive high-quality, safe dental services from professionals and organisations that are competent and meet national standards, and that services improve. Members include: CQC, DHSC, GDC, NHSE. The work is underpinned and supported by: NHS BSA, HWE and the local Healthwatch network.

Scottish Qualifications Authority (SQA) The Scottish Qualifications Authority is the executive non-departmental public body of the Scottish Government responsible for accrediting educational awards.

Smile Clinic Group (SCG) The Smile Clinic Group is a family of practices throughout the UK.

Please note: these explanations/definitions have been taken from the websites of the specific organisation to ensure accuracy at the time. Accessed 1–20 August 2020.

Other Descriptors

Appreciative Inquiry (AI) Appreciative Inquiry is a strengths-based, positive approach to leadership development and organisational change. AI can be used by individuals, teams, organisations, or at the societal level; in each case, it helps people move toward a shared vision for the future by engaging others in strategic innovation.

Associate Certified Coach (ACC) A coaching credential offered by the ICF. Each level requires a set number of training hours and a number of hours of coaching experience. Associates can build up to the level of Professional and then, the highest level – Master.

Blue on blue A military term for incidents of death or injury resulting from friendly fire. In this context it refers to a complaint by a dental professional about another dental professional. Blue on blue referrals to the GDC are increasing.

Caldicott Named after Dame Fiona Caldicott who chaired The Caldicott Committee's *Report on the Review of Patient-Identifiable Information* in 1997. The Caldicott Principles are fundamentals that organisations should follow to protect any information that could identify a patient, such as their name and their records. Organisations should use the Principles as a test to determine whether they need to share information that could identify an individual.

Continuing Professional Development (CPD) The term used to describe the learning activities dental professionals engage in to develop and enhance their abilities. It enables learning to become conscious and proactive, rather than passive and reactive.

Data Protection Act 2018 (DPA) The Data Protection Act 2018 is the UK's implementation of the General Data Protection Regulation (GDPR). Everyone responsible for using personal data has to follow strict rules called 'data protection principles'. They must make sure the information is: used fairly, lawfully and transparently.

Denplan Excel A certification programme developed by Denplan Simplyhealth for dentists to demonstrate excellence in quality assurance, patient care and communication. It shows how much you value and achieve high standards, and that your practice follows effective processes for complying with these regulations.

Dental Care Professional (DCP) Dental registrant groups, in particularly non dentist registrants. Includes dental nurse, dental hygienist, dental therapist, dental orthodontist therapist, dental technician, clinical dental technician.

Dental Foundation Training (DFT) Dental Foundation Training is a broad-based clinical experience in NHS dentistry. In most DFT posts, one year is spent in an approved dental practice with a trainer who is an experienced dental practitioner. Weekly tutorials are provided by the trainer and study days are organised by the Deanery. Previously known as vocational training.

Educational Supervisor (ES) A trainer who is selected and appropriately trained to be responsible for the overall supervision and management of a specified trainee's educational progress during a clinical training placement or series of placements. Educational supervisors in dentistry work with foundation and vocational trainees in general dental practice.

Foundation Trainee (FT) A dentist who has recently completed dental school and works in an approved NHS dental practice with an experienced dental practitioner as their ES. Training is for one year and a certificate of satisfactory completion at the end of training allows the FT to obtain a performer's list number.

General Dental Practitioner (GDP) A dentist who undertakes the broad range of dentistry within a practice. May provide NHS or private dental care or both.

HTM 01–05 HTM which stands for Health Technical Memoranda is one of several guidance documents in a series of Health Technical Memoranda which give comprehensive advice and guidance on the design, installation and operation of specialised building and engineering technology used in the delivery of healthcare. HTM 01–05 is intended to raise the quality of decontamination work in primary care dental services by covering the decontamination of reusable instruments within dental facilities.

Information Technology (IT) Information technology is the use of computers to store, retrieve, transmit, and manipulate data or information. IT is typically used within the context of business operations as opposed to personal or entertainment technologies. IT is considered to be a subset of information and communications technology. An information technology system (IT system) is generally an information system, a communications system or, more specifically speaking, a computer system – including all hardware, software and peripheral equipment – operated by a limited group of users.

Master Certified Coach (MCC) The highest level of ICF credential for coaches, see ACC and PCC.

NHS Performers List The Performers List is maintained by NHS England in accordance with the National Health Service (Performers Lists) (England) Regulations 2013. It is a list of approved GPs, opticians and dentists who satisfy a range of criteria necessary for working in the NHS.

Nolan Principles The Seven Principles of Public Life outline the ethical standards those working in the public sector are expected to adhere to. They were first set out in the Committee's first report by Lord Nolan in 1995 and they are included in a range of Codes of Conduct across public life. The principles are: Selflessness; Integrity; Objectivity; Accountability; Openness; Honesty; Leadership.

Personal Development Plan (PDP) Personal development planning is the process of: establishing aims and objectives (or goals) – what you want to achieve or where you want to go, in the short, medium or long-term in your career; assessing current realities; identifying needs for skills, knowledge or competence. In dentistry a one-year plan is the most useful. SMART criteria help the plan.

Personal Protective Equipment (PPE) The equipment that protects against cross infection and is worn during dental treatment. It comprises gloves, mask or visor, protective glasses and a protective overall. Precautions resulting from Covid-19 has meant masks must be Filtering Face Pieces grade 3 (FFP3) and fit tested to the individual clinician.

PIES An acronym used within the Forton model. It represents categories of resources: Physical, Intellectual, Emotional, Social.

Professional Certified Coach (PCC) An ICF credential for coaches. ICF offers three credentials: Associate, Professional and Master Certified Coach.

Quality Assurance (QA) Quality assurance is the maintenance of a desired level of quality in a service or product, especially by means of attention to every stage of the process of delivery or production.

SMART SMART is a mnemonic/acronym, giving criteria to guide in the setting of objectives. The letters stand for: **S**pecific, **M**easurable, **A**chievable, **R**elevant or **R**ealistic, **T**imely.

Training Programme Director (TPD) A dental training programme director is a member of the Dental Training Committee who is managerially responsible to the Postgraduate Dental Dean for the delivery of dental foundation training within a geographic area.

Vocational Dental Trainee (VDT) The equivalent of FDT in England. VDT's work in Scotland.

Vocational Training (VT) This is required for dental graduates in Scotland and is the equivalent of foundation training in England, Wales, and Northern Ireland. New or recent graduates from UK dental schools must satisfactorily complete a one-year programme of Vocational Training in order to be eligible to hold a Health Board list number. The aim of Vocational Training (VT) in dentistry is to enhance clinical and administrative competence and promote high standards through relevant postgraduate training so as to allow participants to meet the needs of general dental practice.

Further Reading

Alred, B., Garvey, G., and Smith, R. (1998). *The Mentoring Pocketbook*. Management Pocketbooks. ISBN: 9781906610203.

Briggs, A., Clark, J., and Hall, I. (2012). Building bridges: understanding student transition into university. *Quality in Higher Education* 18: 3–21.

Brooks, J.A. (2015). *How to Develop Your Career in Dentistry*. Wiley Blackwell. ISBN: 0001118913817.

Brooks, J.A. (2017). *How to Survive Dental Performance Difficulties*. Wiley Blackwell. ISBN: 978-1-119-25561-1.

Burgo, J. (2015). *The Narcissist You Know: Defending Yourself Against Extreme Narcissists in an All-About-Me Age*, 1–298. New Rise Press.

Clutterbuck, D. (1985). *Everyone Needs a Mentor: Fostering Talent in Your Organisation*. London: CIPD. ISBN: 9781843980544.

Croucher, A. (1998). Burnout and issues of the work environment reported by general dental practitioners in the United Kingdom. *Community Dental Health* 15: 40–43.

Doherty, N. (2010). *Disrupting the Rabblement, the Stockdale Paradox*. Greenleaf book group.

Fenech J., (2013). PIES. www.prezi.com

Gallwey, W.T. (2001). *The Inner Game of Work*, 1–256. Random House Publishing Group.

Hay, J. (2007). *Reflective Practice and Supervision for Coaches*. McGraw-Hill.

Heidari, F., Andrewes, C., Galvin, K. et al. (2002). *Shared Learning and Mentoring for Newly Qualified Staff: Support and Education Using an Inter-professional Approach*. Institute of Health and Community Studies, Bournemouth University.

Hill, R. and Reddy, P. (2007). Undergraduate peer mentoring: an investigation into processes, activities and outcomes. *Metropolitan Universities* 2017 28: 50–66.

Holmes, M. (2012). Spotlight on critical reflection. *Training Journal, Jul 2012*: 1–4.

Hughes, B, Caton Hughes, HR. (2019). No Cape Required: Empowering Abundant Leadership. Business Expert Press (1-177).

Mavin S, Lee L, Robson F., (2010). The evaluation of learning and development in the workplace: Scanning the external environment [Bristol, England]. Higher Education Funding Council for England. pp. 1–30

McKimm, J., Jollie, C., and Hatter, M. (2007). *Mentoring: Theory and Practice*. London: NHSE.

McKinley, N., McCain, R.S., Convie, L. et al. Resilience, burnout and coping mechanisms in UK doctors: a cross-sectional study. *Health Services Research* https://doi.org/10.1136/bmjopen-2019-031765.

McMahon, G. (2017). Dealing with narcissism. *Harvard Business Review*: 1–7.

Richardson, T. (2015). *Walking Inside Out. Contemporary British Psychogeography*. Rowman and Littlefield.

Sansom, L., (2011). Standout Strengths Assessment: A review positive. Psychology News.com.

Schon, D.A. (1987). Educating the reflective practitioner. San Francisco. Jossey-Bass. *Journal of Continuing Education in the Health Professions* 9 (2): 115–116.

Te Brake, H., Eijkman, M., Hoogstraten, J., and Gorter, R. (2005). Dentists' self-assessment of burnout: an internet feedback tool. *International Dental Journal* 55 (3): 119–126.

Thomson N., Thomson, S., (2008). *Working with the Control Influence Accept Model*. www.mindtools.com.

Practical Applications of Coaching and Mentoring in Dentistry, First Edition.
Janine Brooks and Helen Caton-Hughes.
© 2021 John Wiley & Sons Ltd. Published 2021 by John Wiley & Sons Ltd.

Index

Practical Applications of Coaching and Mentoring in Dentistry, First Edition.
Janine Brooks and Helen Caton Hughes.
© 2021 John Wiley & Sons Ltd. Published 2021 by John Wiley & Sons Ltd.